Traditional, Complementary and Alternative Medicine and Cancer Care

Over the last decade, traditional, complementary and alternative medicine has achieved an ever-higher profile amongst academics, healthcare professionals, policy makers and service users, particularly in cancer care. Despite anecdotal evidence of the importance of patient groups and grassroots networks to the way people access therapies, research has tended to focus on the individual.

Traditional, Complementary and Alternative Medicine and Cancer Care provides the first in-depth exploration of the role patient support groups play in the provision of CAM in the UK and Australia. It also looks at the utilisation of non-biomedical treatments in Pakistan focusing on the role of informal social networks.

Drawing on fieldwork in each country, the book explores:

- the empirical, theoretical and policy context for the study of CAM/TM and cancer
- the nature, structure and evolution of patient support groups
- how groups function on a day-to-day basis
- the extent to which what is being offered in these CAM-oriented groups is in any way innovative and challenging to the therapeutic and organisational mainstream
- the ways in which processes of negotiating therapeutic options play out in Pakistan.

Traditional, Complementary and Alternative Medicine and Cancer Care will be of wide interest to those studying complementary and alternative medicine sociologically, to those involved in the provision of cancer care on a day-to-day basis and to those looking to establish a more informed, evidence-based policy.

Philip Tovey is a Reader in Health Sociology at the School of Healthcare, University of Leeds, UK.

John Chatwin is a Research Fellow at the School of Healthcare, University of Leeds, UK.

Alex Broom is a Postdoctoral Research Fellow in the School of Social Science at the University of Queensland, Australia.

For
W. Talist (as always); Betty and Charles
Brian and Alison

Contents

List of illustrations   ix
Acknowledgements   x
List of abbreviations   xi

Introduction   1

PART I   9

1 The empirical, theoretical and policy context in
   international perspective   11

2 Methodology: an overview of approach and
   research sites in the UK, Australia and Pakistan   32

PART 2   47

3 The nature of CAM-focused cancer support groups   49

4 Group performance: enacting therapeutic alternatives
   in the collective environment   65

5 Confined innovation: organisational challenge and
   its limitations   81

6 An exploratory comparative case study from
   Australia   100

PART 3   115

7 Consumption, and perceptions, of traditional,
   complementary and biomedical cancer treatments
   in Pakistan   117

8 Patients' negotiation of therapeutic options   130

9 Interprofessional conflict and strategic alliance   144

   Conclusion   158

   Notes   168
   Bibliography   170
   Index   178

Illustrations

Figures

1.1 Use of traditional medicine for primary healthcare 27
4.1 Layout of the group area 69
6.1 The meditation room 107
8.1 Cancer patients' negotiation of therapeutic options in
Pakistan 134

Tables

1.1 Categories of CAM: National Centre for
Complementary and Alternative Medicine (US) 12
7.1 CAM/TM use and level of education 123
7.2 Use of a *Hakeem* and level of education 123
7.3 Total CAM/TM use by hospital 124
7.4 Socio-economic status by hospital 124
7.5 Perceptions of the effectiveness of TM, CAM and
biomedical cancer treatments 125
7.6 Satisfaction with CAM/TM and biomedical
cancer treatments 126

Acknowledgements

The projects on which this book is based were unusually complex to conduct and a number of people provided invaluable input. Thanks are due to Muhammad Hafeez, Salma Ahmad and Shahin Rashid for their contribution to the work in Pakistan, and to Jon Adams for his involvement in Australia. Thanks are also given to the many people in the UK fieldwork sites who supported the work but who need to remain anonymous; and, of course, we are grateful to the significant number of individual participants in each of the countries. The work was funded by two grants from the Economic and Social Research Council/Medical Research Council under their Innovative Health Technologies programme.

Finally, many thanks to Kathryn Dewison for reading the final manuscript – bhgaft.

List of abbreviations

CAM   Complementary and alternative medicine
CRUK   Cancer Research United Kingdom
DoH   Department of Health (UK)
ESRC   Economic and Social Research Council (UK)
NHMRC   National Health and Medical Research Council (AUS)
NHS   National Health Service (UK)
RCCM   Research Council for Complementary Medicine (UK)
TCM   Traditional Chinese medicine
TM   Traditional medicine
WHO   World Health Organization

Introduction

The use of non-biomedical therapeutics and the management of cancer are high profile issues in health internationally. They both generate, in their own right, considerable debate amongst academics, practitioners and the wider public. Increasingly, as non-biomedical approaches have become more and more a feature of the range of therapeutic options available to cancer patients, the two have become inextricably linked. This book is concerned with that increasingly evident combination. Specifically, it is a socially located analysis of previously under-researched aspects of this coming together in both richer and poorer countries – namely, the UK, Australia and Pakistan.

The book is written at a time of considerable change. In richer countries the entrenched oppositional positions of less than a decade ago are being replaced by a (largely) rhetorical consensus on integration. For many in policy-making arenas the virtues of this trend have achieved an almost taken-for-granted quality in a short space of time. At a global level a seemingly positive shift in attitudes towards the promotion of traditional medicine (TM) as a means of satisfying unmet health need (WHO 2001), and the theoretical possibility of the spread of non-indigenous practices to poorer countries have also established a dynamic of change.

Given these significant and fast-moving shifts in the use of non-biomedical medicines for cancer care it is not surprising that research in the area is at a relatively early stage. While this paucity of research is beginning to be addressed in richer countries (e.g. Bishop and Yardley 2004; Cassileth and Vickers 2005; Ernst and Cassileth 1998; Lewith *et al.* 2002; McClean 2005; Morris *et al.* 2000; Rees *et al.* 2000), beyond the West, research has been minimal. However, as the need for research has become increasingly recognised (House of Lords 2000), two inter-related elements have informed that push: first, the necessity of evidence on the effectiveness and efficacy (as well as safety) of specific practices; and second, the need for 'results' that will inevitably and immediately lead to policy development and practice change.

When researching and writing on any issue within the broad field of 'health' there is an understandable tendency to seek solutions: to fast-track the process of gathering information in order to argue a case for change at whichever level. This is, of course, not specific to health. However, the issues presented by people's suffering, by the persistence of an unequal access to resources which have an immediate and apparent consequence in terms of day-to-day wellbeing, and indeed survival itself, make the pursuit of policy as the logical outcome of each and every study all the more understandable.

And when the health topic in question is cancer, with all its symbolic, and indeed, physical and practical importance and impact, the need to work towards better patient outcome becomes all the more pressing. In the West the expansion of use of non-biomedical approaches has occurred largely in the absence of a biomedical-type evidence base and in a socio-political context of patchy and minimal regulation. In poorer countries, given the global spread of biomedicine, other practices generally exist in a similar context. There are certainly very real issues to address here, such as providing the best available evidence about practices as a means of underpinning informed choice by cancer patients.

However, having acknowledged this, it is crucial to appreciate that there are dangers associated with the development of a narrow policy and practice-driven research agenda. It is naïve to assume that the production of evidence produces, in a simple, deterministic way, a given set of behaviours and decisions amongst practitioners or patients. This is something that needs to be borne in mind across the board in an area as contentious as non-biomedical practices. In the context of non-biomedical practices for cancer, consideration of the multifaceted nature of evidence and legitimacy is absolutely imperative. Positions that have evolved in the absence of an evidence base have been established on the basis of very powerful influences: professional identity, differentiation and jurisdiction claims, ideological affinities, divergent conceptualisations of the nature of disease and so on.

Consequently, there is a need for a very different research agenda to be pursued in tandem with the one rushing headlong towards evidence collation and yes/no policy judgements about the incorporation or isolation of specific therapeutic practices. This is an agenda directed primarily at the generation of an understanding of processes underpinning action. It is a sociologically informed approach which takes its primary purpose to be gaining insight into this social phenomenon as an end in itself. It is not that such work may not, in time, inform health policy and practice; it is rather that it need not be its primary and immediate goal. Indeed, the removal of the 'recommendations imperative' will help to permit the production of focused work which does not have to be spuriously stretched to reveal the supposedly 'generalisable' on the basis of single pieces of work. It will allow the gradual production of a more solid knowledge base which will make for more effective policy making in the long term.

It is against this background that the study(ies) which provide the basis for this book were developed. The studies may justifiably be regarded as either three separate studies conducted in different countries, or as component parts of one broad enterprise. This is because while on the one hand, there are inevitable points of conceptual linkage across the fieldwork sites, on the other hand the specificity of context (as well as method and research questions) makes direct comparison inappropriate. Indeed the analysis presented here should not be seen as comparative in any strict sense. Instead, it should be seen as providing insights into the processes surrounding the utilisation of non-biomedical practices for cancer care in specific locations. Needless to say, especially when setting Pakistan alongside the UK or Australia, the practices used differ greatly and the histories associated with them are similarly disparate. Moreover, while conceptual linkage across countries was manifest in our general interest in, for instance, decision making or the role of advocates of non-biomedical practices, there were also country-specific agendas which needed to be pursued – agendas which necessitated the utilisation of, at times, differing methods, used to collate different types of data.

Thus, the overall purpose of this work was to approach the study of the global phenomenon of the utilisation of non-biomedical treatments for cancer from a fresh angle – to generate types of data and a form of understanding that had not previously been established. There was no attempt to conceptualise this as a means of generating a complete understanding of all aspects of the processes involved. Rather the aim was to engage with country-specific issues in their own terms – issues which in each nation had not been researched before.

In the UK (and Australia) our focus was on group-level action in grassroots patient support groups involved in the advocacy and/or provision of complementary and alternative medicine (CAM) to people with cancer. Born of a recognition that support groups incorporating some form of non-biomedical therapies had proliferated in recent years, but that we had little or no understanding of how they functioned in relation to the provision of CAM, our focus here was on how such groups evolve and function and how their location (frequently on the boundaries of orthodoxy) impinges on those processes. Our approach was deliberately focused rather differently to those studies that have generated data and interpretations of individual CAM use in the West. It was an attempt to balance what has become, arguably, an overly individualised approach to the topic.

In Pakistan, the research questions, though with some overlap, had a very different quality. In part this was due to the inevitably very different socio-cultural circumstances, but it was also influenced by the state of knowledge prior to the study. In this context, although we were primarily interested in how cancer patients negotiate the plurality of therapeutic options available, there was also a need to establish some baseline data on patterns of use. Quite simply there was no previous qualitative work on this topic (as well as virtually no quantitative data). While assumptions could be made about the importance of 'traditional practices' or religion or a range of other things, there was a need to explore these empirically to see if and how such structures and processes were influencing action.

Despite these very real differences, conceptual linkages are evident across the studies. In each case it is the socially located nature of action that is our focus, and while being played out in very different ways, many core themes – the relationship and interaction between biomedical practitioners and non-biomedical practitioners or advocates, the role of evidence, the nature of decision making, etc. – are seen to be cross-cutting themes of importance.

About the book

This book is then based around the findings of the international study introduced above. The book is split into three parts. The purpose of Part 1 is to provide an overview both of the area under study – the use of non-biomedical approaches in the treatment of cancer – and to provide more of an insight into the nature of what was an unusually complex study to conduct. As well as setting up the main empirical parts of the book it is intended that the material drawn together here will be of interest and use in its own right.

In Part 2 we present the findings from the part of the research conducted in richer countries – primarily the UK, but also, as detailed in the final chapter, Australia. It focuses directly on the structures and processes of cancer support groups. Due to the nature of the study, this can both be read as a stand-alone analysis of the nature of such groups in these countries and as part of the broader whole.

Part 3 deals directly with the research conducted in Pakistan. Again these chapters can be read as stand-alone analyses of various issues relating to the mediation of therapeutic options in that country, although inevitably, there are conceptual linkages with Part 2 which will become apparent.

More specifically, the book breaks down as follows. In Chapter 1 we provide an overview of the empirical, theoretical, and where relevant, policy context for the study of CAM/TM and cancer. While inevitably we focus particularly on those countries that form the core of the book (UK, Australia and Pakistan), we also draw on work from elsewhere in the world where this is relevant. During the discussion of Pakistan we include a profile of the broader character of the country which sets out core elements of its economic, social and religious profile. As will become apparent, an understanding of such contextual factors is essential to gaining insight into health-related processes.

Given the conduct of fieldwork in three countries, and the utilisation of different methods between the UK and Australia on the one hand and Pakistan on the other, it is important to detail the approach taken and the elements of context that are specific to each country. This is the focus of Chapter 2. In relation to the UK arm of the study, we pay particular attention to describing the history and character of the eight support groups in which fieldwork took place. As will become evident, although they shared some characteristics, they differed on quite important dimensions. For example, they differed in their relationship with state-provided medical institutions, which, it emerged, is crucially linked to the ways in which CAM provision is operationalised. With the example of Australia, the nature of the single case study is similarly described. For various reasons, both practical and methodological, the approach taken to data collection differed considerably in Pakistan. Given the need to establish a baseline quantification of what was happening on the ground, a survey was conducted before the core qualitative part of the study. The nature and purpose of both parts of the work in Pakistan are explained.

Chapter 3 opens Part 2 and addresses some fundamental issues about the nature, structure and evolution of patient support groups. Within a broader discussion of the groups we argue that two important processes can be identified. First, that a useful differentiation can be made between Type 1 and Type 2 groups. Although clearly an ideal type, this differentiation underlines not only the self-evident differences in history and affiliation of groups, but, rather more interestingly, the influence that this exerts on the evolution of those groups and the place of non-biomedical practices within them. And, second, we outline how groups of both type follow similar patterns of evolution and move through recognisably similar stages. Again, of course, this conceptualisation allows for variation within broadly identifiable processes.

Having opened with a broad analysis of group form and character, in Chapter 4 we focus on the detail of how groups function on a day-to-day basis. We do this through the use of a case study of one particular site. While not intending to present this case as 'representative' in any strict sense, it does provide an interesting point of access into the kinds of issues that have resonance beyond this individual group. The chapter is based around an in-depth look at how a routine meeting of the group is enacted. Amongst the key themes of the chapter are: the tensions that can arise between location and the operationalisation of therapies, and secondly, the role and impact of new members and the mediation of information. We thus consider both structural and interactional elements of the group.

In the final chapter focusing solely on the UK, Chapter 5, attention is turned to an examination of the extent to which what is being offered in these CAM-oriented groups is in any way innovative, and indeed, challenging to the therapeutic and organisational 'mainstream'. We examined this issue because the rhetoric of difference, of providing and being something distinct, is central to the *raison d'etre* of many such groups. We consider, in turn, the nature of formal and informal gatekeeping and how this affects group composition; the actual organisation of the groups themselves; and the extent to which groups offer challenge to broader inequalities. Central to our analysis is a recognition of the 'confined' location (both therapeutic and geographical) within which the groups evolve and function.

Part 2 of the book concludes with Chapter 6. In this chapter attention is shifted to Australia. Here we present findings from a single exploratory case study of a support group in New South Wales. Through an examination of the regular patterns of the group we argue that, in order to identify the value of the group to its participants, we not only need to look at its formal level of operating but also its informal processes. By looking to this informal level, a different mode of activity is identifiable – one which is in many ways freer, due to the absence of the constraints that act on the coordinators of the 'timetabled' meetings. In this informal arena, the exchange of information and ideas frequently takes on a more radical edge, a context which can be seen as facilitating a fuller expression of the priorities of the members rather than reflecting a political judgement on the appropriateness of practices.

Chapter 7 is the first of three chapters looking solely at the study data generated in Pakistan. In order to establish the context for later discussions, this chapter concentrates on the results of a survey conducted with cancer patients in four hospitals in Lahore. Two findings in particular stand out from this initial part of the work. First, that despite the theoretical possibility of the globalisation of non-indigenous CAMs, it was indigenous traditional practices that figured heavily in the therapeutic practices of cancer patients. And second, that there is a need to recognise that traditional medicine is not simply a monolithic category – patients make very different judgements about different individual practices so classified. The latter finding in particular is fundamental to the more detailed analysis of the following chapter.

In that chapter – the eighth – we examine the accounts of cancer patients in Pakistan, generated through one-to-one interviews, in order to work towards an understanding of the actions and attitudes quantified earlier. Specifically, we discuss the process of negotiating therapeutic options by individual patients – but crucially we do so taking full account of their social, cultural and material contexts. We argue that individuals are far from simply and uncritically utilising what is traditional or local. Instead they are actively mediating therapeutic possibilities by drawing on, and at times being constrained by, personal, social and cultural resources. We argue that this can be conceptualised by an appreciation of individuals' active engagement with three temporally and spatially specific dimensions: structural/practical constraint; pragmatic experimentation; and cultural identity and religious affiliation.

The focus of Chapter 9 is on Pakistani cancer patients' experiences of the interprofessional dynamics associated with the range of traditional and biomedical cancer treatments. In this chapter we move away from patients' perceptions of particular treatment modalities, and towards an analysis of their experiences of the dynamics between different therapeutic modalities. A significant theme in this chapter is the apparent existence of considerable differentiation in the dynamics between different traditional modalities and the biomedical community. We examine the existence of strategic alignments between certain traditional healers and the biomedical community, demonstrating a complexity at the interface of TMs and biomedicine in Pakistan. We argue here for the need for a multifaceted understanding of the social and cultural processes underpinning the dynamics of these relationships.

We conclude with a chapter which summarises the key points of the book and draws together its various component parts. We will identify points at which it is useful to establish conceptual linkage between various settings, although we argue that it is important to retain a sense of 'difference' and not impose any artificial unity on the processes described. In this concluding section we also take the opportunity to return to a broader discussion of the value of sociological work in the field which is not tied to immediate and narrow policy objectives. In this context we sketch out an agenda of research priorities for the field.

Part I

Chapter 1

The empirical, theoretical and policy context in international perspective

In this chapter we outline the various empirical, theoretical and policy issues that are crucial for contextualising the studies examined in this book. Broadly speaking, this chapter is split into two main sections. The first section examines issues related to non-biomedical cancer treatments in the UK and Australia (complementary and alternative medicines). The second examines issues related to the use of non-biomedical cancer treatments in Pakistan (mainly, although not exclusively, traditional modalities). Given that these are such different socio-cultural and economic settings (UK and Australia versus that of Pakistan), in this chapter we address the specific issues related to each context separately, preparing the ground for an analysis that emphasises the socially and culturally specific nature of cancer patients' engagement with non-biomedical treatments.

To provide the reader with an overview by which to frame the discussions in the following chapters, we will outline: the nature of cancer services offered in each social context; rates of mortality and morbidity; existing cancer policies; and previous research on use of CAM and TM by cancer patients. Moreover, at a more theoretical level we engage in debates about how to define different healthcare practices and lastly, critically examine existing sociological theory that is relevant to the analysis presented in the following chapters.

Defining healthcare practices

We begin with some consideration of terminology. There has been considerable debate as to whether one should use complementary, alternative, non-orthodox or traditional to describe non-biomedical treatments, and what connotations these categories engender. In recent times the most common label in the academic literature has been 'complementary and alternative medicine' (or CAM). In health policy, and particularly cancer policy, 'complementary' has generally been preferred as it is not suggestive of a set of modalities that offer real alternatives to biomedical treatments. Politically, representing therapeutic modalities like reiki or acupuncture as contributing to, rather than competing with, biomedical care, has seen comparatively less resistance from the biomedical community. Broadly speaking, as summarised by the American National Centre for Complementary and Alternative Medicine in Table 1.1 below, CAM is generally seen to encompass a broad range of practices including such things as: herbal medicine, acupuncture, homeopathy, dietary principles, spiritual practices, hypnosis, osteopathy, chiropractic and so on.

However, whether these practices are complementary, alternative or in fact 'mainstream' is often contested (Eskinazi 1998). Debate about what is complementary/alternative or conventional/orthodox has been amplified by the integration of certain CAM techniques by medical practitioners (see Dew 1997) and the increasing integration of CAM practitioners into biomedical settings. Fuller (1989) has argued that certain so-called non-orthodox modalities such as chiropractic, osteopathy and acupuncture have aligned themselves with biomedicine, muting their metaphysical

Table 1.1 Categories of CAM: National Centre for Complementary and Alternative Medicine (US)

Alternative medical systems	Alternative medical systems are built upon complete systems of theory and practice. Often, these systems have evolved apart from and earlier than the conventional medical approach used in the United States. Examples of alternative medical systems that have developed in Western cultures include homeopathic medicine and naturopathic medicine. Examples of systems that have developed in non-Western cultures include traditional Chinese medicine and Ayurveda.
Mind–body interventions	Mind-body medicine uses a variety of techniques designed to enhance the mind's capacity to affect bodily function and symptoms, including meditation, prayer, mental healing and therapies that use creative outlets such as art, music or dance.
Biologically based therapies	Biologically based therapies in CAM use substances found in nature, such as herbs, foods and vitamins. Some examples include dietary supplements, herbal products and the use of other so-called natural therapies (for example, using shark cartilage to treat cancer).
Manipulative and body-based methods	Manipulative and body-based methods in CAM are based on manipulation and/or movement of one or more parts of the body. Some examples include chiropractic or osteopathic manipulation, and massage.
Energy therapies	Energy therapies involve the use of energy fields. They are of two types: 1) Biofield therapies are intended to affect energy fields that purportedly surround and penetrate the human body. The existence of such fields has not yet been scientifically proven. Some forms of energy therapy manipulate biofields by applying pressure and/or manipulating the body by placing the hands in, or through, these fields. Examples include qi gong, reiki and therapeutic touch. 2) Bioelectromagnetic- based therapies involve the unconventional use of electromagnetic fields, such as pulsed fields, magnetic fields, or alternating-current or direct-current fields.

overtones in an attempt to increase their compatibility with the biomedical model. It is argued that this process of assimilation has been exacerbated by professionalisation and in particular the establishment of qualifications, licensing and regulatory bodies in certain alternative modalities (Saks 1998). These developments have disrupted dichotomous representations of CAM and biomedical practices. This has resulted in various attempts to justify practices as 'alternative', 'complementary' or 'conventional' in accordance with access to state funding, access to insurance rebates, those accepted and used by the public, those condoned by the medical community and so on (e.g. Eskinazi 1998). However, these criteria are limited, as they are rapidly changing and are inconsistent internationally. Further, there is no agreement amongst social commentators as to what level of insurance coverage, or degree of state funding must be met before a profession is considered 'conventional', notwithstanding the problem of multiplicity within particular modalities.

There are similar issues with what to call what many people refer to as 'Western' or 'modern' medicine. Historically, Western medicine (insofar as this is even a valid category in itself) has been referred to as 'modern', 'conventional' or even 'traditional'. However, these categories have obvious limitations (particularly with the increasing presence of indigenous 'traditional' medicines) and thus within the following chapters we generally refer to Western medicine as *biomedicine*. This category of biomedicine, we argue, is a less loaded term in that it merely refers to the ideological basis of the practices we generally recognise as 'modern' medicine (i.e. techniques based on the application of the principles of the natural sciences and especially biology and biochemistry), rather than suggesting its progressiveness (i.e. modern) or geographical roots (i.e. Western).

Despite the aforementioned ambiguities, there are certain things we can say about the character of what is generally referred to as CAM and TM, and the features that tend to delineate CAM and TM from biomedicine. CAM generally refers to healthcare practices not offered systematically by biomedical organisations in richer, Western countries (Zollman and Vickers 1999). Many CAM practices are derived from traditional health practices, but over time they have adapted to (and been shaped by) Western models of care (e.g. herbalism, reiki or naturopathy). Certain CAMs, which have their origins in traditional belief systems, have moved away from the belief systems on which they were originally based (e.g. Chinese acupuncture), resulting in different, but not completely distinct, healthcare modalities (e.g. Western forms of acupuncture). Other CAMs have emerged within Western culture (i.e. homeopathy) but are distinct from biomedicine in terms of the paradigmatic basis for their treatments. Thus, although encompassing a disparate range of modalities, what largely characterises CAM is a lack of integration into Western healthcare systems (Kelner and Wellman 1997), and second, their tendency to espouse models of care which incorporate (or at least give reference to) physical *and* metaphysical elements in treatment processes (however, this is not true of all CAMs). Such CAMs are ubiquitous across richer countries and there is anecdotal evidence that suggests that they are beginning to achieve a presence in poorer countries too. There is, therefore, some merit in identifying them as 'globalised CAMs' – in distinction to localised TMs.

Traditional medicine (TM), in this context, refers to local knowledges, belief systems and therapeutic practices that are used in poorer countries (and in some cases, within richer countries by ethnic minorities and indigenous peoples) for health-related purposes. Whereas CAMs have historically (at least, over the last century) operated on the periphery of most Western healthcare systems (although this is slowly changing), traditional medicines have often been the dominant means of treatment for health problems for centuries (e.g. traditional Chinese medicine in Chinese society), and in some cases, they continue to dominate healthcare beliefs and practices. Traditional medicine, as a category, is thus characterised more by longevity, cultural specificity, religiosity and having indigenous roots (WHO 2001), than by its position relative to other modalities (as has been the case for CAMs). Moreover, paradigmatically, there is no clear pattern in the ideological basis for TMs, whereas for CAM, a case could be made (although problematic) for a degree of congruence in the ideological positioning of many complementary and alternative health practices.

Cancer in the United Kingdom

In order to set the context for an examination of CAM use by cancer patients, it is useful to reflect first on the social and economic impact of cancer in the UK and Australia. Each year in the UK more than 275,000 people are diagnosed with cancer and the number of people diagnosed each year is increasing (CRUK 2006). The biggest risk factor for cancer is age, and given the UK's ageing population, there is little doubt that there will be increasing rates of morbidity over the next few decades. There are more than 200 different types of cancer, but breast, lung, large bowel and prostate account for over half of all new cases. Cancer is the cause of more than a quarter (26 per cent) of all deaths in the United Kingdom, with 154,547 people registered as dying from it in 2003 (CRUK 2006). While cancer accounts for an increasing proportion of deaths in the UK, cancer mortality rates have dropped by 11 per cent over the last ten years. There have been large falls in the mortality rates for cancers of the cervix, stomach, bowel, lung and breast, which when combined account for 45 per cent of deaths from cancer in the UK. The main reasons for falls in mortality are the primary prevention of cancer, earlier detection and better treatment (CRUK 2006). Breast cancer is the most common cancer in the UK despite the fact that it is rare in men.

Lung cancer is still by far the most common cause of male death from cancer, causing a quarter of all male cancer deaths. In 2003 there were 19,806 deaths from lung cancer in men in the UK (CRUK 2006). Prostate cancer is the second most common cause of cancer death in males, accounting for 13 per cent of the male deaths from cancer in 2003. Over 92 per cent of deaths from prostate cancer occur in men aged 65 and over (CRUK 2006). For women in the UK, there are similar numbers of deaths from lung and breast cancer. In 2003, lung cancer was the most common cause of death, responsible for 13,630 deaths in women compared with 12,614 deaths from breast cancer. Deaths from breast, lung and large bowel cancer together account for nearly half (46 per cent) of all female deaths from cancer (CRUK 2006).

While other richer comparable European countries report similar rates of morbidity from cancer, there is evidence to suggest that, for many cancers, survival rates are lower in the UK (see Department of Health 2000). For cancers like breast cancer and bowel cancer, this is partly because patients tend to have a more advanced stage of the disease by the time they are treated. The DoH suggests that this is probably because: patients are not certain when to go to their GP about possible symptoms; GPs have difficulty identifying those at highest risk; and because of the time taken in NHS hospitals to progress from the first appointment through to diagnostic tests to treatment (2000). Furthermore, the DoH acknowledges that the variation in quality and provision of services across the country means that not all patients are getting the optimal treatment for their particular condition. It suggests that decades of under-investment in people and equipment have taken their toll on the NHS cancer services, and it has come under increased pressure to adopt new ways of working and fully exploit new treatment methods to keep NHS cancer services at the forefront of international progress (see Department of Health 2000). Equipment, it would seem, is out of date and is often incapable of delivering state-of-the-art procedures for diagnosis and treatment, and the NHS has too few cancer specialists of every type. For example, the United Kingdom has around eight oncologists per million population, less than half that in other comparable European countries (Department of Health 2000). And there has been a failure to modernise services by adopting new ways of treating patients.

Cancer in Australia

In Australia, more than 88,000 new cases of cancer are diagnosed each year (The Cancer Council Australia 2006). One in three men and one in four women will be directly affected by cancer before the age of 75 and more than half of them will be successfully treated. The survival rate for many common cancers in Australia has increased by more than 30 per cent in the past two decades, but over 36,000 people die from cancer each year. The most common cancers in Australia (excluding non-melanoma skin cancer) are colorectal (bowel), breast, prostate, melanoma and lung cancer (The Cancer Council Australia 2006). Cancer costs AUS$2.7 billion in direct health system costs (5.7 per cent) and AUS$215 million was spent on cancer research in the year 2000 – above 18 per cent of all health research expenditure in Australia (The Cancer Council Australia 2006).

Cancer incidence in Australia is higher than in the United Kingdom and Canada, but lower than in the United States and New Zealand. However, Australia's mortality rates are lower than all four of these countries (The Cancer Council Australia 2006). The melanoma incidence rates in Australia and New Zealand are around four times higher than those found in Canada, the UK and the US. However, mortality rates for melanoma in Australia are quite low compared with other countries. Australia's mortality rate for lung cancer is significantly lower than that of the US. For men, the mortality rate is 32 per cent (lower than the US) and 48 per cent for women (The Cancer Council Australia 2006). Incidence of colorectal cancer in Australia is higher than that of the UK, the US and Canada, but less than that of New Zealand. Australia's mortality rates for colorectal cancer are also high by world standards, including above those of Canada, the UK and the US (The Cancer Council Australia 2006).

CAM and cancer in richer countries

General interest in CAM therapies has grown at an exponential rate (Cant and Sharma 1996), and the use of CAM in relation to cancer treatment and palliative care is acknowledged as being particularly widespread. Significant numbers of patients now combine their biomedical cancer treatment with some form of CAM (Richardson et al. 2000), and Ernst and Cassileth (1998) report that, on average, around 31 per cent of all cancer patients use some form of 'unconventional' therapy. UK surveys have shown similar figures with over 30 per cent of people with cancer reporting use of CAM (Lewith et al. 2002; Rees et al. 2000). In a recent study, Scott et al. (2005) surveyed 127 adult patients with a diagnosis of cancer from both Scotland and England. CAM use was reported by 29 per cent of the sample. The use of relaxation, meditation and the use of medicinal teas were the most frequently used therapies. A study by Harris et al. (2003) of 1077 Welsh cancer patients found that 49.6 per cent of participants had used at least one type of CAM during the past 12 months and 16.4 per cent had consulted a CAM practitioner.

Various quantitative surveys have indicated that CAM is also frequently used by Australian cancer patients (e.g. Miller et al. 1998; Salminen et al. 2004; Sibbrett et al. 2003). Salminen et al. (2004) surveyed 156 Australian cancer patients and over half the patients (52 per cent) had used at least one 'unproven' therapy since their diagnosis, and 28 per cent had used three or more. Sibbrett et al. (2003) completed a survey of 9375 Australian women aged 73–78, and found that, for all cancers combined, 14.5 per cent of women had consulted an 'alternative' practitioner. This percentage varied depending on the type of cancer: skin (15 per cent), breast (11.5 per cent), bowel (8.8 per cent), and other (16.5 per cent). In their study of 215 Australian breast cancer patients, Salminen *et al.* (2004) found that 17 per cent used 'supportive' and 'complementary' therapies. Therapies tried by patients included visits to a naturopath (11 per cent) and use of herbal preparations (8 per cent).

Although more research is needed to confirm such trends, studies also suggest differentiation according to patient characteristics. For example, in a study of Canadian women with breast cancer, Boon *et al.* (2000) found that 67 per cent of breast cancer patients use CAM therapies – significantly more than that reported for many other patient groups. Morris *et al.* (2000) investigated the hypothesis that use of CAM therapies differed between patients with breast cancer and those with other primary tumour sites (N = 617) and found that breast cancer patients were far more likely to be consistent users compared with those with other tumour sites, suggestive of variability between patients with different types of cancer. Further research has shown that gender mediates decisions to use CAM amongst cancer patients, and that the wealthier middle classes are more likely to access non-biomedical treatments (Thomas *et al.* 2001). However, despite significant variability across patient groups, it would seem that in general, cancer patients are significant users of CAM. In total Australians currently spend around $1.8 billion of private money a year on CAM and CAM therapists (see MacLennan *et al.* 2006).

This high proliferation of CAM within a relatively defined area of healthcare – an area that in fact often embodies cutting-edge biomedical developments – has meant that the conflicts, misalignments and power struggles that underlie much of the biomedical/CAM dynamic are likely to be even more visible. Consequently, along with the general trend towards greater practitioner awareness of CAM, there have been calls for oncologists in particular to make themselves aware of the kinds of CAM therapies that patients are likely to come across as they progress along the trajectory of their illness. Cassileth and Chapman (1996), for example, propose that oncologists need to work on providing an environment in which patients can feel comfortable talking about CAM treatments.

Active collaboration between CAM and biomedicine is currently extremely limited, and this may be one factor that continues to generate a sense of mistrust between professional groups. Advocates of CAM often regard biomedicine as actively resisting the increased role of complementary medicine. As a result, critiques of CAM based on notions of efficacy and safety put forward by biomedicine are often interpreted as purely attempts to maintain a position of power and control (e.g. Chapman-Smith 2001). The apparent reluctance of many biomedical physicians to become involved with CAM at anything other than a superficial level (they may be happy to refer patients to therapists for, say, massage or relaxation even if they do not practise CAM therapies themselves), does little to quell such concerns.

There are also pragmatic and professional reasons why contact between CAM and biomedicine may be restricted. It is currently not a legal requirement – in the UK at least – for many types of CAM practitioner to undergo training before advertising their services (Stone and Matthews 1996), and until recent moves towards more biomedical forms of professionalisation and self-regulation among many CAM disciplines (e.g. Cant and Sharma 1996), it was not uncommon to find CAM practitioners without any formal training at all. Similarly, there are problems of consistency which significantly complicate attempts to define CAM. As suggested earlier in this chapter, complementary and alternative medicine is not a single unified system of medicine but a vast array of practices and therapies, few of which share a common philosophy or principle (British Medical Association 1993). In their Survey of Knowledge and Understanding of Unconventional Medicine in Europe, the Research Council for Complementary Medicine (RCCM), for example, listed 60 different CAM therapies (RCCM 2000). Even the ideals and causal underpinnings of therapies that have established a well-codified theoretical base can cause difficulties. Some forms of CAM, such as homeopathy, are fundamentally polarised with respect to the biomedical paradigm, and this limits the degree to which a useful dialogue with the biomedical community can be generated.

The arena of cancer care in particular has become resonant with increasingly vocal calls for openness and integration in relation to CAM. This may reflect an acknowledgement within the medical profession that when faced with a life-threatening illness for which biomedicine often holds little hope of cure, people are likely to be interested in the possibility of help from any quarter, regardless of whether or not it is sanctioned by the biomedical community (Revil 2002). Ernst (2000) evokes an image of many cancer patients as '... desperate individuals who understandably want to leave no stone unturned' (p.307). Similarly, Salmenpera et al. (1998) highlight the abundant evidence suggesting that cancer patients' proclivity for CAM treatments does not always stem from a hope that they will produce miracle cures, but is more often seen simply as a practical means of counteracting the unpleasant side effects of biomedical cancer therapies. The much cited report on the state of CAM research in the UK for the Science & Technology Committee of House of Lords (2000) painted a similar picture, focusing on those 'safe' and well-established therapies that are beginning to be incorporated into parts of the NHS: acupuncture, aromatherapy, massage, healing, etc., each representing forms of CAM that have adopted professional guidelines prohibiting practitioners from claiming that their systems can 'cure' cancer.

Health policy and CAM in cancer care: UK and Australia

The high demand for CAMs amongst UK cancer patients, and recent politi-cal pressure for a more integrative approach to cancer (House of Lords 2000), has led to developments in cancer policy that, albeit implicitly, attempt to promote a more diverse, integrative and patient-centred approach to cancer care (e.g. Department of Health 2000; Department of Health 2001; Tavares 2003). Albeit sporadically, CAM services are now being provided to selected cancer patients within some National Health Service (NHS) hospitals and NHS-affiliated hospices in the UK. These organisations are offering selected CAM therapies including (but not lim-ited to) reiki, reflexology, aromatherapy, therapeutic massage, spiritual healing, acupuncture and hypnotherapy. These have generally been the 'healing' and 'touch' CAM therapies due to perceptions of their 'benign' and 'uncontroversial' nature.

However, despite some progress towards a more open approach to can-cer care, policy calls for integration are still rigidly centred on the creation of a biomedical-type evidence base as key for progress to occur (e.g. House of Lords 2000). UK policy makers are thus caught between reinforcing the existing trajectory towards evidence-based medicine (EBM) in the context of CAM, and the growing realisation that an EBM platform may in fact be incommensurable with pursuing an integrative model of cancer care. However, thus far there has been little acknowledgement of, or prepared-ness to engage in, debates about the epistemological and ontological issues that arise in attempts to measure the 'effectiveness' of paradigmatically dis-tinct therapeutic modalities.

The policy context in Australia in relation to CAM and cancer is perhaps even less developed than the UK. Currently there is no formal cancer policy in Australia for the integration of CAM treatments into biomedical cancer care. A recent senate enquiry (including submissions from major cancer stakeholders) recognised the division in Australian cancer care between bio-medical services and complementary and alternative services (see Senate Community Affairs References Committee 2005; NHMRC 2005). Among other recommendations, this report emphasised the need for clinical prac-tice guidelines to help ensure that cancer patients can discuss their interest in complementary therapies with healthcare professionals in an open and non-judgemental way, and second, that more work should be done on pro-viding efficacy data on commonly used 'unproven' treatments (Senate Community Affairs References Committee 2005). As part of this report the Senate Committee recommended that the National Health and Medical Research Council (NHMRC) appoint two representatives (including one consumer) with a background in complementary therapies, to be involved in the assessment of research applications received by the NHMRC for research into complementary and alternative treatments (Senate

Community Affairs References Committee 2005). The purpose of this was the attempt to counter perceived biomedical bias in reviews of CAM-related research proposals submitted to the NHMRC – a perceived barrier to producing more evidence on the efficacy of CAM in cancer care and thus further integration. Although it remains to be seen what impact this report will have, if nothing else, it illustrates increased political pressure for formalising the role of CAM in cancer care in Australia.

The sociology of CAM

The sociology of CAM is an area of enquiry that is both young, theoretically underdeveloped and empirically underinvestigated (Siahpush 1999; Tovey *et al.* 2003; Chatwin and Tovey 2004). In the 20 years or so since the field began to become a recognisable entity in its own right, much work has been concerned with positioning it within the context of biomedicine and wider social trends, and examining the motivations and reasoning behind the apparent upsurge in interest. The importance of research that incorporates the perspectives of lay culture(s) as well as those of the medical (and CAM) community has also been emphasised from early on (Kronenfeld and Wasner, 1982). In tandem with studies aimed at providing definitive information about developing CAM usage, patient and practitioner motivations and beliefs, etc., there has also been work seeking to unravel issues of legitimation, professional dominance and agency. Within this strand of investigation the 'medical' aspects of CAM become relatively incidental, and issues of proof and efficacy are similarly marginalised. Sharma (1993), for example, has been concerned with defining the anthropological and sociomedical context within which CAM should be approached, highlighting what she described as a collective uncertainty over where the new discipline should lie and how it should be approached. Early work by Fulder (1992) was similarly aimed at grounding what had hitherto been a relatively diffuse arena, and as the field became more defined, the dynamics of professionalisation and integrational conflict between CAM therapies and biomedicine have attracted attention. This has mainly centred on specific therapeutic traditions. Cant and Sharma (1996), for example, were concerned with the progression towards professionalisation followed by homeopathy in the UK, and examined the ways in which claims for legitimacy, status and authority can be linked to the presentation of homoeopathic knowledge. A similarly therapy-based focus was taken by Briggs (1989) in relation to chiropractic developments in Canada. Miller (1998) focused on the professional identity of osteopaths, while Boon (1998) analysed the world views of naturopathic practitioners, and how the conflict between their holistic and scientific socialisation informed their practice behaviour.

There seems to be as yet, however, little sociological investigation into the dynamics of more extreme and newly coalescing (in terms of professionalisation and structured organisation) forms of CAM in the UK (Chatwin and Tovey 2004). Some studies have focused on the situation in other countries, both richer and poorer, however, which may inform the situation in the UK and Australia. Ngokwey (1989), for example, made connections between diagnostic specificity and definitions of the 'healer' role in three faith healing institutions in Brazil. Similarly, Lindquist's critique of the 'culture of charisma' surrounding healers working in contemporary urban Russia (Lindquist 2001) demonstrates how devices of legitimation (such as the appropriation of religious imagery) are crucially dependent on cultural references – something, which again, might readily inform an analysis of the situation in the UK and Australia.

Complementary and alternative medicine has also been located within broader social theory. Rayner and Easthope (2001), for example, position its rise within a postmodern paradigm and highlight the way in which the features that have come to define CAM (in terms of its commodification) – such as its development into niche markets and the promotion of lifestyle values – can be seen as accurately reflecting features predicted by theories of postmodern consumption (see also Featherstone 1991). One of the first writers to describe the commodification of the value systems associated with much CAM was Coward (1989). She argued that a 'new consciousness' was emerging that challenged many of the taken-for-granted assumptions of the Western world, the elements of this new consciousness being a preference for the 'natural' over the scientific and technical, a rejection of expertise, an increasing awareness and concern about risk, a moral imperative to take responsibility for one's actions and, coupled with this, a prioritisation of personal choice.

There has also been some empirical work focused on examining Coward's theoretical position in relation to CAM. Siahpush (1998, 1999), for example, used a small-scale telephone survey of residents in the Australian town of Albury-Wodonga to evaluate the differential influences of what he described as 'postmodern values' on attitudes towards 'alternative' medicine. The research was later expanded into a follow-up study in Victoria (Australia), and incorporated dissatisfaction with medical outcomes and dissatisfaction with the medical encounter. Siahpush found that the postmodern values of a preference for the natural, rejection of the technical and so on, were associated with a positive attitude towards alternative medicine, and in the second study, he was also able to identify trends towards belief in responsibility for one's own health, and holistic views on health. Significantly, in neither study was dissatisfaction with medical outcomes or of the medical encounter a major factor. Rayner and Easthope's study (2001) moved beyond the abstract concept of alternative medicine and concentrated on a concrete indication of its use – the purchase of alternative medicines. Interviews with 100 purchasers of alternative medicines at a variety of outlets (i.e. biomedical chemists, health food shops and a homoeopathic chemist) indicated that purchasers could be roughly cate-gorised into two main groups. The first group did not hold the postmodern values posited by Coward (1989); they tended to value expertise and did not demand personal choice. They generally purchased 'generic' prepara-tions such as evening primrose oil or herbal medicines. The second group, who were likely to purchase homoeopathic and aromatherapy products, were committed to holism, choice and control of their lives. It is this second group – that was generally younger than the first – that appeared, according to Raynor and Easthope, to hold 'postmodern' values.

There are points of compatibility between postmodern theory and the approach taken by Tovey and Adams (2003) in their exploration of CAM and nursing. Tovey and Adams (2001) argued that a neglected sociological theory, social worlds theory (developed within the tradition of symbolic interactionism – Strauss 1978), provides both tools and structure that are well suited to the sociology of CAM. This theoretical framework introduces notions of authenticity, appropriation, legitimacy to the sociology of health professions (Tovey and Adams 2003). These have direct applicability to everyday CAM practice and the study of it. Tovey and Adams asked such questions as: has nursing an essentially authentic relationship with CAM? If so, why? And at the expense of whom? How and why is the appropriation of therapies (by nursing) occurring? And with what legitimacy? They found that CAM was used as a method of distinction and professional legitimacy within certain sub-worlds of nursing, and that such processes were not lin-ear. Other parts of the nursing profession were opting to reject the validity of CAM and draw on the biomedical model (and alliance with biomedical clinicians) as a means of reinforcing professional legitimacy.

Adopting an anti-determinist 'social worlds' perspective, their emphasis is on fluidity, both in the variety of data that define an actor's 'social world' – in this case the social world of the nurse using CAM – and also in the con-textualisation of these data. Actor and context are seen as constantly shifting, reshaping and reacting. The fundamental unsuitability of tradi-tional social theories being applied to the study of non-biomedical treatment use has been highlighted by Alder (1999), and it seems that in this context, the social worlds approach is ideally suited to the investigation of CAM because it can effectively mirror the holistic environment it is engaged in analysing (see also Chatwin and Tovey 2004).

There is also a body of work on professional power and legitimacy in the context of the relationship between biomedicine and non-biomedical treat-ment modalities (e.g. Broom 2002; Norris 2001). Such analyses have focused on the hegemony of biomedical organisations in consistently sidelining other treatment modalities which challenge their occupational control over primary care. Arguments have centred on the deployment of restrictive notions of efficacy and evidence that are pervasive in the health-care policies of the UK and Australia. Much attention has been given to the impact of the EBM movement and other evidence-based trajectories in limiting the scope of health services and the potential integration of paradigmatically disparate treatment modalities. Such issues have emerged as increasingly important given that there is significant questioning of such policies even within the medical fraternity. This has led sociologists to increasingly question the role of ideology in maintaining occupational control and delimiting movements towards a more integrative form of healthcare (e.g. Mykhalovskiy 2003; Pope 2003).

A further strand of investigation that has emerged recently is the application of micro-interactional methodologies – most notably conversation analysis (CA) – to the arena of CAM consultations. From its early development out of ethnomethodology in the late 1960s and early 1970s, CA has been rigorously applied to the analysis of the structures of talk that occur within medical interactions (Heritage and Stivers 1999; Drew *et al.* 2001). The objective is to map those routinely occurring interactional behaviours that serve to define and perpetuate, for example, unequal power relationships between patient and practitioner; or the idiosyncratically asymmetrical environment that medical talk engenders. One of the main commonalties of CAM therapists is that they tend to seek to empower patients through more egalitarian communication practices (Chatwin and Tovey 2004).

The interactional misalignments that can occur therefore, as hitherto marginal therapies seek to develop more conventional professional standing, while at the same time remaining true to their holistic principles, are of particular interest (Chatwin and Tovey 2004). Comparative analysis of complementary and biomedical encounters at a micro level can describe precisely those activities that cause most 'trouble' for patients and practitioners, but which may be hidden beneath the noise of interactional familiarity and convention. Similarly, and perhaps more usefully, it can also help to map the intricate and ostensibly unconscious reciprocal positioning that generates helpful and therapeutic medical encounters. It appears that very little micro-interactional work has been carried out specifically in the area of oncology consultations, but as the degree of CAM integration into the mainstream grows, the need to understand the interactional dynamics of the arenas identified by broader ethnographic work will demand a greater application of these micro-interactional tools.

The internal dynamics of such systems at a professional level, and the interrelationship between them and biomedicine, are also relatively unexplored (Chatwin and Tovey 2004). Similarly, and of more direct relevance, a key feature of much of the work in this field has been a polarisation between the individual and the individualised consumer and practitioners (Adams 2000). There is currently little understanding of the decision making, network and information utilisation and negotiation involved in the pathway to CAM (Siahpush 1999) in the context of support groups; the 'group' is under-represented at the expense of the individual. It is for this reason that in the first empirical chapters of this book we examine the group as an entity which is involved in the construction, mediation and definition of CAM and how it is experienced by the individual.

CAM and support groups

Along with the traditional supportive role that patient support groups have come to play in cancer care, it is evident that they are also having a major (although as yet largely unresearched) influence on the engagement of cancer patients with CAM therapies. Active participation in such groups (and not necessarily ones that advocate CAM) has been found to have a positive psychological function for many cancer patients (Targ and Levine 2002). A study by Montazeri *et al.* (2001), for example, is typical in finding a correlation between group involvement and improved psychological wellness amongst breast cancer patients. Similarly, Michael *et al.* (2002) found that cancer rehabilitation programmes benefit from the availability of social support networks. Involvement in such support groups, however, has also been shown to have possible drawbacks, for both patients and their carers. Damen *et al.* (2000) interviewed members of a cancer support group in Belgium and found discrepancies between the generally positive image of such groups propagated in academic and official literature, and the personal views of group members. Similarly, at a functional level, Fulton *et al.* (1996) describe how involvement in a group can undermine or restrict previously established lines of support, and how members often develop a form of 'reality' relating to the ongoing experience of their situation. This necessarily creates a degree of experiential separation between them and other relevant parties, such as professional carers. In practical terms, this might translate into building up a repository of knowledge about complementary therapies as they relate specifically to a certain oncological condition (Small and Rhodes 2000). Tensions between group members and their biomedical practitioners, many of whom may be hostile towards such therapies, may then emerge. Fulton *et al.* (1996) also suggest that the cultivation of narrow perspectives by certain types of support group is likely to restrict its ability to cater for the needs of potential members.

Connections between the small but significant number of patients who reject biomedical treatments for cancer altogether and the developmental dynamics of some informal and semi-formal support groups may be relevant in informing the investigation of more mainstream organisations. The significant role that such groups can play in supporting the patient when they reject the authority of biomedicine has been explored by Montbriand (1998). The cancer patient narratives that she presents almost universally describe an acrimonious split from biomedical oncology care as explorations of 'gentler' CAM treatments became more appealing. While the focus of Montbriand's study is overtly on oncology patients who wholly abandon biomedicine, and as she herself acknowledges, this group only accounts for around 5 per cent of cancer patients, it again highlights that the need for an awareness of the issues of respect and understanding between patients and their professional carers if irreversible communication breakdowns are to be avoided. It also begins to address important factors related to the development of self-help groups and cancer support groups, in particular those of agency, control and empowerment. Montbriand devotes a small but significant section of her discussion to the way in which the abandonment of biomedical treatment, and the subsequent channelling of a patient's energies into, say, intense dietary regimes, spiritual healing – or in this context, the creation or active involvement in a self-help group – can play a key role in re-establishing a sense of empowerment and control. Similarly, for some, the act of organising their energies in this way can itself become a form of therapeutic activity.

Patient-centredness and patient involvement in the treatment process and decision making are generally assumed to benefit both service providers and patients (Ademsen 2002). Peace and Manasse (2002), in their discussion of the integrated care system established at the Cavendish Centre in Sheffield, highlight an assessment process in which patient involvement plays a key role in the design of individual CAM treatment regimes. Turton and Cooke (2000) have similarly drawn attention to the positive role that empower-ment can play at significant shift points in the trajectory of a patient's understanding and acceptance of their condition, and recommended an approach to cancer care that incorporates this.

On a broader level, issues of patient participation, involvement and empowerment have similarly been closely allied to the development of many small cancer support groups. Empirically, several of the grassroots organisations and informal networks that comprise the case studies exam-ined in the following chapters, for example, have their origins in the experience of a single individual, a trend confirmed by Urben's (1997) Cancerlink survey which found that the majority of cancer support groups were started by someone with cancer, or a relative of someone with cancer. Ademsen (2002) found that the positive effects of participation in small support groups could be attributed to their inherent capacity for universal-ising personal problems, and while pointing out that there is no evidence to indicate that involvement in such groups can extend the life expectancy of members, noted that this was often not their explicit concern. Small and Rhodes (2000) outline how the ongoing and intensely 'lived' nature of much palliative care has made it a field that has lent itself particularly well to the development of these kinds of group. Gott et al. (2002), however, highlight that there can be wide variations between the numbers of groups organised around different types of cancers: citing the Directory of Cancer Self-help and Support (Cancerlink 1998), for example, they contrast 155 listings for breast cancer groups, compared with four for testicular cancer and none for lung cancer.

It is evident that much of the sociological investigation carried out in this arena has tended to focus on those groups that have professional input (e.g. from specialist nurses) (Urben 1997). And while this does account for some 40 per cent of UK cancer self-help organisations (Urben 1997), there are clearly a significant number of groups that are essentially independent and fall more readily into the category outlined by Fulton *et al.* (1996) (Cancerlink 1998; Cancerbackup 2001; Macmillan Cancer Relief 2002). They may, for example, overtly focus on providing something that is fundamentally different from the experience engendered by much of the biomedical cancer treatment process (Montbriand 1998). Michael *et al.* (2002), for example, point to broad elements of positive social integration as being highly significant in the quality of life experienced by individuals once their disease has been diagnosed, and this too is likely to be something that support group membership augments.

The majority of the larger charitable organisations that are involved in the provision of CAM for cancer patients, however, are run along biomedical lines; that is, they regard it as their role to augment and enhance the biomedical model of cancer care rather than to provide an alternative to it. The advocacy of individual therapies in this context can therefore be connected to a large extent by the degree to which therapies have been sanctioned by the biomedical community (the UK's Macmillan Cancer Care and Marie Curie Cancer are examples of this type of national organisation). Smaller organisations that share a faith in 'grassroots' activity (Vincent 1992) and more readily fulfil the definition of a self-help group outlined by Johnson and Lane (1993) (in that they are usually run on a voluntary basis for and by their members) are much more likely to represent a position that questions the relevance of the biomedical model in favour of the subjective reality of the individual's experience (Fulton *et al.* 1996).

In summary, there is a real need to examine the role of the patient support group in the growing popularity and use of CAM for cancer care. In particular, as discussed in the following chapters, support groups play an important (and previously unexplored) role in both the encroachment of CAM on biomedical cancer care and exclusion of such practices.

Non-biomedical cancer treatments in poorer countries

The academic study of non-biomedical healthcare practices has been an essentially Western-based project. Pakistan provides a good example of a country that has hitherto failed to attract an in-depth analysis of its pluralistic medical practices. The country has a long history of support for TM[1] and it is clear that use of TM continues alongside Western-oriented practice. However, there has been very little quantitative research aimed at mapping patterns of use, and there has been no sociological work designed to flesh out these statistics or position them within a cultural paradigm for which many of the semantic and social assumptions applied in the West may not be appropriate.

International healthcare policy and traditional medicine (TM)

Global health organisations such as the WHO are putting increasing emphasis on the importance of traditional health systems for poorer countries (Bodeker *et al.* 2005). Recent policy trajectory has been towards a melding of traditional and biomedical systems, with a focus on the accessibility and affordability of traditional health systems (WHO 2001). It would seem that policy makers are increasingly acknowledging the vital role traditional medicines will play in reducing excess mortality and morbidity in poor and marginalised populations (see Bodeker *et al.* 2005). Moreover, traditional medicines are viewed, in some cases, as more culturally attuned to local needs and belief systems. Use of TMs in many poorer countries is considerable, as shown in Figure 1.1. However, there is a paucity of sociological research examining patient decision making in relation to different modalities, and specifically, how local values and belief systems may influence treatment choices.

In poorer countries, health practices have often been inextricably linked to religious or spiritual belief systems. In fact, in many countries religious figures also act as health advisers, with disease often linked to religious or spiritual powers. Although many poorer countries are increasingly embracing biomedicine, there still exists close connections between prevailing religious beliefs and some traditional healthcare systems (see Tovey *et al.* 2005).

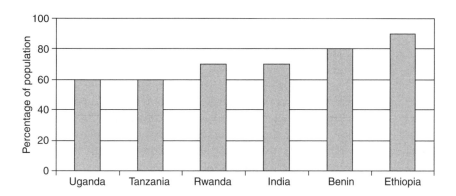

Figure 1.1 Use of traditional medicine for primary healthcare
Source: WHO 2001

The social, political and economic context of Pakistan

With an estimated population over 150 million (UNICEF 2006), Pakistan is the seventh most populous country in the world. Being a largely agricultural country, 67 per cent of its population live in rural areas and about 57 per cent of its civilian labour force are employed in agricultural occupations. Although figures are quite difficult to obtain, 13 per cent of its population were living below US$1 a day between 1992 and 2002 (UNICEF 2006). UNICEF reports that Gross National Income (GNI) per capita in 2003 was US$470 (a rise of only US$70 since 1990). In 1999, the life expectancy for men and women was reported to be 64 and 66 years, respectively. Health services operate on very limited resources, currently about 1 per cent of the GNP (Tovey *et al.* 2005). The public sector provides only 20 per cent of these services, and most people use an eclectic private sector in which healthcare is provided not only by formally trained doctors, but also by pharmacists, paramedical health workers and traditional practitioners of various systems of medicine: *Hakeems, Pirs* and many others (see below for a more in-depth description) (Tovey *et al.* 2005).

Pakistan is a multicultural society with rich social and cultural diversity. The population is predominantly Muslim (96.7 per cent) with a minority of other faiths including Christians, Hindus, Ahmadis, Zoroastrians, Buddhists and Sikhs. Both Urdu and English are the official languages; however, eight other languages are spoken in different parts with different dialects, making Pakistan a multilingual society (Tovey *et al.* 2005). Urdu is understood and spoken almost everywhere and is considered to be the national language. The adult literacy rate (people over 15 who can read and write) amongst adult males in 2000 was 57 per cent and amongst females was 28 per cent (UNICEF 2006). Secondary school education (percentage of enrolments between 1998 and 2002) was 29 per cent for males and for females 19 per cent.

Cancer in Pakistan

There is no population-based cancer registry in Pakistan, so accurate data on the incidence and prevalence of cancer are not available. According to World Health Organization estimates, Pakistan has about 150,000 new cancer cases per year. The total number of patients registered at recognised cancer care facilities is estimated to be between 25,000 and 30,000 per year. This suggests that a large number of cancer patients never reach the Pakistan cancer services. Cancers affecting the largest proportion of the population are female breast cancer, certain lymphomas, leukaemia, cervical, gall bladder and lung cancers (the latter, primarily in men). Significantly, too, for a poorer country, the incidence of colon cancer is high. There is a high frequency of oesophageal cancer around Caspian City, cancer of the mouth in the southern part of Pakistan (attributed to tobacco use) and lymphomas and leukemia in impoverished regions. The facilities that are available for cancer treatment are comparable to well-run hospitals in richer countries. Hospitals have had a major impact on cancer awareness in the regions where they are located, and for those who can access hospital care, patients have access to clinical services in medicine, surgery, medical oncology, paediatric oncology, radiation oncology, nuclear medicine, radiology and pathology. Patients who generally use the state-run hospitals may be referred from throughout the country, but cancer treatment is expensive (even public treatment) and this obviously places limitations on access and availability (Tovey *et al.* 2005).

In paediatric oncology, for example, the average treatment cost of a child with cancer varies from Rs. 75,000 (£800) to Rs. 300,000 (£3,200) (Tovey *et al.* 2005). In richer nations, cancer in children is often curable. In Pakistan, however, most children with cancer die, mainly due to their family's inability to afford treatment. More than 80 per cent of cancer patients in Pakistan need financial support for treatment. For example, because financial support is often unavailable, more than half of those patients diagnosed with lymphoma receive insufficient treatment or no treatment at all.

Traditional medicine in Pakistan

Traditional medicines in Pakistan are multifarious and it is thus useful to differentiate between certain important practices. *Hikmat,* delivered by a *Hakeem* (sometimes spelt *Hakim*), is an approach to the body and illness practised mainly among Muslim communities in South Asia (Tovey *et al.* 2005). A re-organised Muslim development of the system of medicine outlined by Hippocrates and Aristotle, it involves the use of a variety of herbs and minerals. *Hakeems* are generally trained through a process of apprenticeship and usually come from a lineage of healers. However, there is a number of established institutions training people in *Hikmat* in Pakistan (Tovey *et al.* 2005). Recent acknowledgement by the Pakistan government of the value of *Hakeems* has led to the establishment of clinician positions in some hospitals. However, they are considered of lower status and receive lower salaries than doctors.

Spiritual healing, and the practice of *Dam Darood,* are also important forms of traditional medicine. These practices involve prayers, prophetic medicine and other local practices. Such practices are usually delivered by holy men called *Pirs* either personally or through a designee (Tovey *et al.* 2005). *Pirs* will often read verses from the Quran and blow words towards the patient. This process is called *Dam, Dam Darood* or *Dua* (prayer). Another popular form of religious healing is *Wazifa,* which involves multiple repetitions of Quranic verses for weeks or months (Tovey *et al.* 2005).

Levels of TM and CAM use by cancer patients in Pakistan

To date there has been very little research on the use of TM or CAM by cancer patients in Pakistan. The limited quantitative research that has been done on CAM/TM use by cancer patients in Pakistan suggests that, as in the West, TM and CAM use is relatively high (54.5 per cent of all patients). Malik *et al.* (2000) found that traditional herbal medicines (70.2 per cent) and homeopathy (64.4 per cent) were the most commonly employed methods. Thirty-six per cent of the cancer patients employed these methods before receiving any biomedical treatment. Only 15 per cent used these methods after biomedical options had been exhausted. However, the small number of studies that have been done have tended to conflate TM and CAM (i.e. non-biomedical treatments), and second, focus merely on prevalence of usage rather than issues of effectiveness and levels of satisfaction. All were done in Karachi, and none had examined such issues utilising qualitative methodologies. Thus, in our study reported in Chapters 7, 8 and 9, we examine a multitude of issues related to TM and CAM use by Pakistani cancer patients, providing significant insight into patients' relationships with different therapeutic modalities within a pluralistic, and poorer, medico-cultural context.

Conceptualising the role of TM

There has been virtually no work on the sociology of TM and its intersections with biomedicine or CAM. The work that has been done within the social sciences has tended to be anthropological in nature. These projects have included work into traditional healing systems in India (Khare 1996), Thailand (Golomb 1985), Bolivia (Bastien 1987) and Botswana (Haram 1991). Although large segments of this work are quite old, the studies illustrate some key issues that need to be re-examined in contemporary contexts, such as potentially problematic dynamics between (and within) biomedicine and traditional medicine and the strong links between local cultural and religious beliefs and the role, and position, of traditional healers.

In Golomb's (1985) study of traditional healers in Thailand, she found that much more was at stake than the health of the patient when people make decisions about which practitioners (traditional or biomedical) to consult. The choice of a particular kind of medical knowledge was, she argued, just as much a political statement as a therapeutic measure. Moreover, in the socio-cultural context in which Golomb was studying, southern Muslim curers (generally mystics or spirit mediums) provided not only remedies for health problems but also guidelines for maintaining socio-cultural separatism for the local population from both colonial and other indigenous groups. Thus traditional healers played a wider part in the social fabric than merely as health advisers.

Khare (1996) found that the therapeutic pluralism evident within Indian culture impacts significantly on the delivery of biomedical care. For example, the vast majority of biomedical Indian doctors routinely learn to practise how to treat a patient as much more than a biological and a modern political–legal individual. This trend, it is argued, has emerged from an historical approach to disease and to the person which has close links to traditional therapeutic models. Khare also observed the responses of Indian traditional healers to the increased presence of biomedical interventions, reporting that traditional practitioners are sometimes severely critical of biomedicine and at other times grudging admirers. Khare observes that *Hakeems*, as we observe within the Pakistani context (see Chapters 7, 8 and 9), often view biomedical care with significant negativity, or as he reports, 'like a cage that separated a patient from his relatives, home and even his own self' (p.844).

Napolitano and Flores (2003) examined the ways in which the 'traditional' was deployed (and translated) as a means of negotiating foreign forms of modernity (i.e. biomedicine) in South America. Moreover, they explain the popularity of traditional medicine as related to the emergence of a new citizenship or empowerment of the individual (particularly in the context of difficult living conditions) (Napolitano and Flores 2003).

In Bolivia, Bastien (1987) documented how traditional healing systems and mythologies could be utilised to educate biomedical practitioners on how to communicate biomedical knowledge with local populations. In this way, paradigmatically disparate healing systems were combined as a means of addressing health concerns amongst a socially and culturally specific (and historically mythological rather than physiological) population.

Whereas anthropological research into TM has focused on religious and cultural identities of local and indigenous populations and the impact of 'modern' science on local belief systems, we were interested in extending this to questions raised in the sociology of CAM. Because of global changes in the time since these studies and the growth of sociological study of non-biomedical practices, we thought that the area could benefit from being studied from a different angle. This meant engaging with TM in relation to issues often examined in the sociology of CAM, including: patterns in patient perceptions of effectiveness; beliefs about the legitimacy of 'science' or 'holism'; and the impact of interprofessional disputes about patient care.

Chapter 2

Methodology

An overview of approach and research sites in the UK, Australia and Pakistan

In this chapter we outline the various methods used to collect the data presented in the rest of this book. As suggested in the introduction, in one sense this book utilises data from a range of different research projects; however, these projects are also inextricably linked in terms of the insights they provide into decision making with regard to non-biomedical healthcare practices. As illustrated below, the approaches used in the three different countries shared certain commonalities but also differed in important respects. The information provided is intended to help make sense of the data presented in subsequent chapters. As such, as well as details of process, we pay particular attention to outlining the nature of fieldwork sites: namely, the user groups in the UK and the hospitals (and their geographical context) in Pakistan.

The UK arm

In order to achieve an in-depth, focused understanding of user groups – their histories, objectives, and their day-to-day functioning, as well as their intersection with related networks, practices and organisations, we need a multi-dimensional means of data collection. Consequently, here we used a case study approach. We selected eight discrete patient support groups. Although it would have been inappropriate to try to establish a definitively 'representative' corpus, our selection was based on the need to reflect the broad spectrum of organisations most commonly encountered by cancer patients. As will be shown, while these groups are at first sight quite different in make-up, location and so on, they also have similarities which cut across organisational form – not least in the tendency to provide rather similar forms of CAMs to be accessed by their members.

The process of selecting our eight core case study sites began with an extensive search of the resources that most NHS cancer patients would have access to. Thus, at a broad level, we utilised the comprehensive directories of UK CAM/cancer support organisations provided by Macmillan Cancer Care (Kohn 1999), and Cancerbackup (Cancerbackup 2001), along with internet sources, and leads generated as we established deeper contacts with key players in the field. From an original list of around 60 potential groups, 16 were short-listed. These were then narrowed down to eight, the key criteria for inclusion being that they must be involved in offering some form of CAM – be this simply at the level of providing information about treatments, or actually facilitating the practical provision of such therapies. In order to reflect more readily the actual make-up of the field (i.e. the fact that it extends from the relatively 'mainstream', right through to the marginal and obscure), groups were not selected on the basis of the types of CAM they championed. Rather, the fact that they had any degree of CAM involvement rendered them eligible for inclusion. The main criteria for non-inclusion at this stage were the practical limits of access; understandably, initial enquiries at some groups revealed that the kind of in-depth semi-ethnographic approach we were taking was perceived to be too intrusive or too demanding in terms of involvement for participants. Similarly, in some of the more esoteric and essentially 'outsider'-oriented groups that were approached, there was a definite sense that they felt we might be trying to undermine them – to 'prove' that what they were doing was either pointless or dangerous. This, as we found out once fieldwork was under way, was a sense of caution which influenced other aspects of group functioning. The eight case study sites which were finally confirmed reflected a mix of varying sizes and resources, rural/urban positioning, gender basis and cancer types. This selection also reflects variations in size, location (urban and rural), affiliation (i.e. NHS and independent), different cancer types, funding sources, membership levels and so on. In the following section we provide a basic outline of the characteristics of each site.

The UK case study sites

Site I

This site is run by a single CAM therapist (a 'natural healer'), and although it is technically 'independent' (see Chapter 3), it operates from within the organisational structure of a standard NHS cancer hospital. It has been established for around 15 years, and concentrates mainly on the provision of relaxation and meditation. Its approach is overtly secular, and its membership base comprises patients, carers and other stakeholders (including staff at the host hospital). Individuals not directly receiving treatment at the hospital are welcome to attend meetings, but as the group is not widely advertised outside the hospital, they do not form a major part of the membership. The format for therapy provision is based around weekly meetings which last around an hour. These are held in the hospital and routinely consist of guided meditations. They are facilitated by the main therapist/organiser. Patients who attend the group may also ask for 'one-to-one' sessions with her. These last for up to an hour and are also held within the hospital in a small dedicated treatment room. Referrals to the group come mainly by word of mouth, and via staff at the hospital. Group attendance is fairly fluid, with an average of ten participants regularly taking part in activities.

Site 2

Site 2 is a medium-sized nationally recognised organisation. It was founded in 1980 with the objective of pioneering a holistic approach to cancer care. The group claims to be an 'acknowledged leader in the field of holistic cancer care' and provides a wide range of CAM-based therapies on a short-term residential basis (the organisation operates from a single location). Courses and treatments are open to patients and carers/supporters, and the emphasis is on integrating with, and supporting, the biomedical treatments that patients may be taking. The organisation is charitably funded and receives clients from all over the UK and abroad.

Site 3

This site is a very small, rural cancer support group operating on a charitable basis. It has been established for around seven years and is based in a community arts facility which forms an integrated part of a much wider community health and welfare initiative. Not originally set up with a specifically CAM agenda, the provision of therapies is now taking on a more central role. Very much a 'local' group, membership is relatively static, and recruitment limited to a small number of hospitals, GP surgeries and clinics. The main function of the group is to provide a central meeting space where people can make contact, obtain information and participate in group activities related to cancer care. CAMs on offer are supplied on an *ad hoc* basis by private therapists from the local community. Most activities are offered at a reduced rate or for free. At the time of fieldwork, these included massage, art therapy and aromatherapy. Meetings are held once a month, and routinely attract between five and ten participants. The group has an active circle of non-attending members (mainly friends and relatives of patients) who fund-raise and perform administrative duties.

Site 4

Site 4 is a small CAM-oriented support group based in a holistic medical centre in an urban location. The group is relatively new, having operated for only two months at the onset of fieldwork. It holds monthly meetings which may be attended by anyone who has cancer and an interest in CAM/holistic treatments. Carers and supporters are also encouraged to attend. Meetings are organised around overtly holistic principles, with an emphasis on non-hierarchical leadership and facilitation. In this sense, the meeting itself is designed to have a therapeutic impact, but specific CAMs are also on offer, including homeopathy, massage, t'ai chi, herbal medicine and art therapy. These are provided by a core team of organisers who are largely drawn from the medical centre which hosts the group. Routine group attendance is between eight and 15 participants.

Site 5

The aim of site 5 is to 'offer a programme of healing for the whole person, working at all levels of the mind, body and spirit' (quoted from group advertising material). In this sense, the organisation is overtly aimed at providing the facilities for a wide range of CAM modalities to be offered and practised. It still, however, operates as a distinctly 'conventional' or 'mainstream' support group in that members can utilise meetings simply to socialise and make contact with people in a similar position. The group originated in 1989, meets twice monthly, and has a very well established place in regional cancer care. It is a charitable organisation run by a large group of volunteers from a variety of backgrounds (with a strong emphasis on recognised qualifications for any CAM therapists who become involved). Routine attendance at meetings can be over fifty.

Site 6

Site 6 is a well established NHS-affiliated hospice with charitable status. Because of the environment in which it is based, it tends to have a high turnover of members (which are almost exclusively drawn from the hospice). Therapies on offer include aromatherapy, massage and relaxation. These are provided 'in-house' by nursing staff who are trained therapists with (NHS) recognised CAM qualifications, although local CAM providers are occasionally hired on an *ad hoc* basis. Site 6 does not operate formal group sessions as such, but is more a loose affiliation of providers offering services as and when they are required as part of palliative cancer care. The underlying hospice environment provides an overall structure and identity for members and therapists.

Site 7

As an internet forum dedicated to discussions on CAM treatments for prostate cancer, site 7 is essentially a virtual support group. It is facilitated by a single patient who monitors the large number of 'posts' which appear daily. Membership is not limited to cancer sufferers, and a proportion of individuals who take part in the various topic threads which develop are carers and health professionals. As with many internet-based forums, people who wish to post messages are required to register before taking part, and usually take on some form of pseudonym as a user name. Similarly, a number of rules and conventions are placed on members relating to their conduct on the site. The forum is officially based in the US, but a significant number of members originate from the UK.

Site 8

Our final site is a well established group based in an NHS hospital. It serves a large metropolitan area and draws its membership from a range of other regional NHS and private cancer service providers. Originally a purely biomedically orientated support group offering social and information services, site 8 has now been supplying CAM-based therapies and activities for around five years. Modalities on offer include art therapy, t'ai chi, relaxation classes, aromatherapy, massage and healing. These are provided as an adjunct to the routine support functions of the group. As an organisation with strong NHS connections, therapists engaged in providing CAM for members are required to be 'suitably' qualified, and are subject to stringent vetting procedures. Along with offering CAM-based activities, site 8 also acts as a central hub for a variety of smaller local support groups.

Data collection

In this UK arm of the research, we utilised three main sources of data collection:

1   Interviews (informal and semi-structured)
2   Analysis of documents
3   Observation of meetings and day-to-day processes.

Interviews

The purpose of utilising semi-structured and informal interviews was to achieve an understanding of varying conceptualisations of CAM, the different meanings it has for people, and its place in the (social) management of cancer. We also wanted to explore how CAM impinges on notions of cancer as a disease, ideas about the effectiveness of treatments, and how its role may influence the development of personal control over treatment processes.

Interviews were conducted with a wide range of stakeholders (patients, group administrators, practitioners, etc.). In order to obtain a wide spread of perspectives, no restrictions were placed on which individuals connected with a group were approached, and recruitment of participants was routinely snowballed (Gilbert 1996: 73) from an initial contact with a main organiser or facilitator. This person provided an all-important first contact through whom it was possible to legitimise approaches to other members. Connections, and subsequent interview opportunities, tended to emerge from here. This approach was informed by an understanding of patient groups or charities as embedded in a web of other groups and networks, and as constantly evolving through intersection with them. Interview recruitment at any given group was continued until saturation was achieved; that is, until the process was adding nothing new to our understanding of that particular organisation.

Interviews were qualitative and semi-structured or informal in nature. This enabled us to adapt to the myriad of positions and perspectives that were in evidence. The themes of the interview schedules were continually reviewed (and revised as necessary on the basis of emerging evidence), and were individually tailored to the situation of each interviewee. We explicitly pursued negative cases as a means of enhancing the validity of our propositions as they developed. There were, however, a number of thematic elements which were addressed in every case. These were:

1   The individual's basic demographic information
2   Their relationship to, or role within, the group (i.e. organiser, regular member, fund-raiser, CAM therapist, etc.)
3   Their experiences with cancer that had led them to be involved
4   The history of their illness and treatment
5   If they organised a group, or worked as a CAM therapist, how they came to be involved in the group
6   Their perspective on CAM and their understanding of the various therapies they encountered (or provided)
7   Their views on CAM in cancer care, and their personal experiences of its use in their particular group context
8   Lastly, we wanted to explore issues directly related to group functioning and group dynamics. How was the group they were involved in actually organised? Were there tensions or problems with its functioning, and how did it fit into wider healthcare networks?

These themes formed the basis for the majority of interviews, although again, the specifics of individual cases and their particular relation to a given group often meant that the interview formats that were actually used differed quite widely between participants. In all, we conducted over 50 interviews across the eight case study sites. These were audio-recorded where possible and transcribed verbatim. Analysis of transcription data was conducted alongside ongoing analysis of data from our other main sources.

Document analysis

Our analysis of relevant documents allowed us to establish an understanding of the priorities and agendas of groups and served to contextualise the findings generated from other sources of data. These data ranged from publicity material and formal documentation pertaining to an individual group's activities, right through to audio recordings, information CDs and DVDs produced by these organisations. The importance of documents varied according to the size and scale of the case study group, and selection of material was informed both by our initial research questions and by the information that emerged during the course of ongoing fieldwork. However, we were deliberately eclectic in our definition of what we considered to be relevant as we wished to obtain as complete a picture as possible of the context within which stakeholders developed a perception of the groups they encountered.

Document analysis also helped us to examine the ways in which support groups presented themselves to potential members, and how they displayed (direct or indirect) alignment with given positions on CAM. At another level, we were able to utilise reports, accounts and other media to gain an understanding of the practicalities of group functioning – how written and recorded information underpinned the fabric of activities. For any given group, we identified all formal expressions of intent/policy statement relating to the use of CAM, with particular emphasis on drawing out models of health and illness which underpinned statements, positions on professional/lay relations and so on. We also collated broader documents that impinge on CAM as a discrete therapeutic and socio-medical area. In larger charities this included overall policy aims, and elsewhere, policies relevant to those networks, practices and organisations which impinged on the functioning of the groups (CAM nurses, hospitals that housed a support group, etc.). Lastly, where possible, we identified any relevant 'series' of documents: reports from meetings at which CAM issues are discussed.

Observational work

Observational work was of considerable importance to this project. However, the actual form that this took was influenced by the nature of the case study group. The day-to-day functioning of some organisations meant that direct observation of activities was not practical or relevant; the internet-based discussion group (site 7), for example, was obviously precluded from this type of investigation. In most cases, the approach taken was one of participant observation; the researcher actually contributing to the activities that were taking place – generally as a 'lay' member of the group. In the context of cancer support and CAM, this position is reconciled by the fact that most groups actually encourage carers, friends, and lay members to attend. Very few groups (and none in our corpus) restricted the attendance of people without an experience of cancer. Similarly, the 'nature' of the CAM activities which routinely crop up in the cancer support group environment are not routinely reliant on all participants actually being ill. As we shall explore, it is a singularly egalitarian feature of CAM that it can enable sufferers and non-sufferers to participate together in key therapeutic activities. The actual observational work carried out therefore varied from group to group. It ranged from sitting in on small-scale t'ai chi and meditation sessions, through to non-participant observation of administrative meetings at larger organisations. Again, we were conscious that the observable and relevant aspects of a group's functioning could extend well beyond those discrete activities enacted at 'formal' meetings. We were keen to obtain data from 'around' the environments within which groups were embedded – particularly those operating out of biomedical settings (i.e. groups which were based in NHS environments such as cancer hospitals). These included 'satellite' encounters, such as those that might be enacted between group members and non-group healthcare staff. The observation of interactions of this nature helped clarify interrelational aspects of CAM/biomedicine dynamics, and allowed us to compare the reported perspectives of group members (as relayed in interviews, etc.) with direct observations of ongoing behavioural dynamics.

The Australian study

The Australian section of our work represents a self-contained exploratory study, but one that was designed to provide material that would fit directly with, and complement, the UK and Pakistan data. Australia, as a richer country, is in many ways similar to the UK. As with the UK, however, virtually no empirical data exist on the role that cancer support groups and networks play in providing CAM services. We also hypothesised that the socio-medical structure in Australia (a mix of private and public health provision) may have an impact on the ways in which cancer support organisations are arranged, and in particular, how they engage with and mediate CAM.

Method

In order to provide a useful counterpoint to the other two arms of the project (UK and Pakistan), an in-depth case study approach was taken. Due to time restrictions and other logistical considerations (the fieldwork was limited to one month), it was decided that resources should be concentrated on investigating a single relatively 'mainstream' cancer support organisation. A colleague in Australia helped identify a suitable group, and much of the pre-planning and organisation for the trip (including gaining local ethical approval in Australia) was done in advance.

This case study approach was designed to match the methodological approach we also used in the UK (as outlined above). We aimed to find out about the overall make-up of the support group, the nature of the members, including their interests and backgrounds. Much like the themes we explored in the UK arm, we were interested in how they perceived the role of CAM in their cancer care; the group's position as part of a biomedical cancer hospital; the dynamics of its location within the Australian socio-medical paradigm; and the extent to which participants with knowledge of other groups saw processes here as reflecting broader trends. To this end we again collected data in three ways:

1   Qualitative interviews, both informal and semi-structured, with group organisers, group members and other stakeholders. Due to a certain compatibility of socio-cultural context, we were able to utilise broadly the same thematic format as that adopted in the UK (see above). In all we conducted interviews with seven regular group members, and with the two facilitators who ran the group.

2   Document analysis, including the collection of publicity material by and about the group, reports, policy/intent statements, group hand-outs and other documentation. In this particular group we were fortunate to have access to the regular internal evaluation question-naires which the facilitators utilised to canvas the opinions of the group participants – a source of data which was not available for any of the UK case studies.

3   Lastly, like the UK arm, we utilised participant observation of group activities. In this case, this involved the researcher taking part in three of the regular (weekly) meetings which the group held, along with the infor-mal pre/post-meditation interactions within which these activities were embedded. The group meetings took the form of structured meditation sessions, and were particularly suitable for participant observation.

A brief description of the Australian case study group is given below. The structure and origins of the group are discussed in more detail in Chapter 6.

Study site: the meditation group

The Australian group is based at one of three large public hospitals that serves a coastal region in NSW. This hospital is primarily known locally as a centre for oncology services and offers a range of auxiliary and support services for cancer patients and their carers, including occupational therapy and genetic counselling. Within the hospital grounds is a hospice which pro-vides pain and symptom management, short-time respite care and terminal care. The cancer support group located at the hospital was chosen as a case study site from a shortlist of five possible CAM/cancer groups in the NSW area. The main reasons for its inclusion included: its relatively small size made it amenable to a concise period of fieldwork; its provision of CAM was straightforward (i.e. it ostensibly focused on providing only one activity – meditation); its client base was largely drawn from the local area, which would simplify the logistics of interviewing group members; it was structurally positioned within a biomedical health setting, providing an interesting comparison with similarly positioned UK groups; and was considered by local informants to share many characteristics with user groups elsewhere. Importantly too, the group was known to meet on a weekly basis, which allowed for a number of participant observation sessions to be incorporated into the month allocated for fieldwork.

The Pakistan arm

Whereas the UK and Australian arms of this study were qualitative in nature, our work in Pakistan utilised both qualitative and quantitative methodologies. At the outset of the study there was virtually no data available on the use of TM or CAM in Pakistan and we considered it important to map out wider patterns of use before conducting a more in-depth qualitative analysis. Initially, therefore, we completed a quantitative survey of cancer patients before moving on to conduct in-depth interviews.

Quantitative method

Our quantitative data corpus involved a structured survey of cancer patients in four different hospitals in Lahore, Pakistan. To give an idea of the context of Lahore, it is a city of over 7.5 million people and is positioned 25 kilometres from the border with India. It is the second largest city of Pakistan and a hub of economic activity. Major industry situated in the district includes foundries, steel mills, textile units and chemical factories (Government of Lahore 2006). Lahore is considered the cultural capital of Pakistan and has the largest number of educational institutions in the country.

We took our sample from four hospitals in Lahore which had the following characteristics:

Hospital I

This is a 450-bed government teaching hospital. Treatment is free for government employees but private patients have to pay for their treatment. If they cannot afford to pay they seek help from local charities or from the personal resources of the doctors. The catchment area is not fixed and patients come from all areas of Punjab.

Hospital 2

This is an 80-bed government cancer hospital with no fixed boundary for its catchment area. However, it is mostly patients from Lahore and its suburbs who come to this specialist cancer hospital for treatment. Treatment is not completely free but rather is means-tested on an individual basis. However, government employees get free treatment.

Hospital 3

This is a government teaching hospital but treatment is free only for government employees. Private patients have to pay for treatment and those who cannot afford to pay get assistance from charitable organisations operating in the hospital. Patients from all over Punjab come to this hospital.

Hospital 4

This is a 25-bed private hospital treating patients from all areas of Pakistan and sometimes Afghanistan. Treatment costs are expensive for those who can pay but those who cannot are given free treatment or partial help with treatment costs.

The decision to draw our sample purely from the four aforementioned hospitals was made due to the centralisation of cancer-related health facilities in Lahore, rather than in rural parts of the Punjab province. Because of this centralisation of health services, the majority of cancer patients in the Punjab province come to Lahore for treatment (thus providing a fairly representative sample of the whole province).

The survey was carried out between April and August 2003.

Sample

We had no prior knowledge about the proportion of patients that would be users of CAM/TM within the studied population, so we took as a conservative estimate for the population proportion of the cancer patients having access to CAM/TM in and around Lahore to be half. Furthermore, we decided that the sample estimate of this proportion to be accurate to within 0.05 (precision of the estimate) at 95 per cent confidence. The resulting sample size was 385 patients. Working with this figure, it was decided that we would aim to survey 350 to 400 cancer patients over a four-month period. It was decided that the respondents/patients would be distributed among the four hospitals according to the bed capacity of their cancer wards. All the hospitals treated cancer patients from different parts of the province/country; however, the specialist cancer hospital had the most diverse geographical representation of patients. All 362 patients approached during these times completed the survey.

Fieldwork

Before the survey was conducted the medical and research directors of the hospitals were approached for permission to undertake the study and all subsequently gave permission. Two male and two female researchers undertook the survey, which took place in the oncology department of each hospital. Each of the four researchers had training in survey methods and were sociology graduates. Generally the male researchers surveyed the male patients and female researchers the female patients, but at times, female researchers surveyed male patients as well. When recruiting began, researchers would report on a daily basis to the hospitals' management to ensure the appropriate authorities were aware of their presence and knew that the study was being conducted. The researchers approached all patients admitted to the hospitals during weekdays – on different days and at different times of the day (between 10:00 and 16:00) until the predefined number of surveys for each hospital was reached. The researchers gained informed consent from the patients before the survey was completed. The patients were told that they were being interviewed as part of a survey to seek information about their disease and treatment behaviours. Usually patients had one or two family members/carers with them while the survey was being completed. A large number of patients from one hospital took part in the study as it had a large number of cancer patients. The interviewers themselves filled in the questionnaires, not the patients.

Qualitative methods

The qualitative Pakistan data came from semi-structured interviews, following the quantitative survey, with 46 cancer patients in the same four hospitals in Lahore. Participants in the first survey were asked whether they would also be prepared to take part in a semi-structured interview. Most of the 362 patients asked agreed. From these we purposively sampled to achieve a spread of ages, gender, cancer types, socio-economic status and stage of disease. Patients were interviewed either in their own homes or in their hospitals. Female interviewers interviewed the female patients, although both female and male interviewers interviewed male patients.

The study (including both the qualitative and quantitative arms) was an unusually complex one to conduct. Funding for the work had been secured from the Economic and Social Research Council (ESRC) in mid-2001. International political events of that year (the destruction of the Twin Towers in New York) dictated that planned visits to oversee the work had to be cancelled, as a consequence local collaborators were identified and data collection was carried out by locally trained researchers and postgraduate students. The interviews were conducted in Urdu, Punjabi or English. They were tape-recorded with the permission of participants and, where necessary, translated into English in Pakistan. This process was monitored by a multi-lingual Pakistani sociologist resident in the UK and transcripts were then sent to the authors in the UK for analysis. Ethical approval was sought and gained by collaborators in Pakistan. Before interviewing began the medical directors of each hospital were approached for permission to undertake the study. Before patients were interviewed we gained written consent.

As with the other qualitative arms of the study, the methodology applied in Pakistan draws on the interpretive traditions within qualitative research, focusing on establishing an in-depth understanding of the experiences of the respondents and, in particular, their accounts of the way they negotiate decisions about available therapeutic options for cancer. Specifically, patients were asked to describe aspects of their decision making processes, including such things as: perceptions of various traditional and non-indigenous treatment options; influence of community and family; the relative importance of cost and geographic proximity in decision making, and so on. Data analysis was based on four questions adapted from Charmaz's approach to social analysis (1990): What is the basis of a particular experience, action, belief, relationship or structure? What do these assume implicitly or explicitly about particular subjects and relationships? Of what larger process is this action/belief, etc. a part? What are the implications of such actions/beliefs for particular actors/institutional forms? One of the authors undertook primary analysis; interpretations produced were challenged and tested by another team member; initial interpretations were re-tested against the data and the final understanding of the data generated.

Concluding comments

The purpose of this chapter has been to provide a concise overview of the main features of the research sites and the principal means used to collect data. The following empirical sections should be seen in the context of the approaches taken and the sites studied. For instance, in the UK our purpose was to throw light on group-based rather than individual action. And while our sample incorporated a range of different sites and thematic consistency was indeed evident, selection of sites using different criteria would necessarily have influenced results. Similarly, the results of our study in Pakistan should be seen both in terms of our regionally specific focus and in relation to the methods used. Our use of one-to-one interviews, for example, inevitably directs attention towards that individual and away from collective forms of decision making. While, as will be seen (especially in Chapter 8), the social location of participants, and structural and cultural influences, are explicitly recognised, adopting a different (say ethnographic, community-based) approach may have produced slightly different emphases. Of course, such work remains to be done.

Part 2

Chapter 3

The nature of CAM-focused cancer support groups

Introduction

In this chapter we will begin to focus in on some of the main issues that contribute to an understanding of how the various types of cancer support group that are involved with CAM in the UK actually work. We will explore the key characteristics of these organisations, and describe how these influence the way they function and evolve. We ask such questions as: what types of people become involved with groups – both as organisers and regular members? In order to contextualise our analysis, we will begin by outlining the larger organisational structures within which various types of support group develop and operate, and how these structures have essentially led to the evolution of two distinctive organisational approaches. We will consider the ongoing and unavoidable influence that paradigmatic tensions between the biomedical community and CAM have had on the way these groups develop and function; tensions which influence everything from access to potential group members, through to the wording used in publicity material. Finally, we will focus more specifically on the role of patients within CAM-based groups and examine their rationales for involvement.

The self-help groups, networks and charities concerned with providing CAM services for cancer patients are eclectic (Kohn 1999). Organisations range from those that are essentially divisions of biomedical healthcare (such as groups based in oncology units or hospices), through to 'grassroots' groups that have no formal affiliation with local health networks. Although the plethora of group types and organisational approaches means that no two groups are exactly alike, and a truly representative data set would be very difficult to obtain, in this study we tried to include a reasonable cross-section of organisations. We concentrated on the most common types seen in UK cancer settings, and which the average cancer patient is likely to encounter as part of their routine treatment journey. Despite wide variations in approach, ethos, funding, membership base and so on, we argue that it is useful to identify two broad umbrella categories of support group. Of course, these typologies are not absolute and points of intersection inevitably occur. However, the differentiation acts as a valuable heuristic device. We have designated them Type 1 and Type 2.

Type I groups

These were essentially established organisations before branching out to provide CAM services. These groups are often formulated along 'traditional' sociomedical lines and the incorporation of selected CAM therapies does not have any significant impact on their organisational direction or ethos. They are routinely affiliated to NHS hospitals or hospices, and are, therefore, likely to have a strong institutional grounding (i.e. they are frequently led or organised by medically trained individuals such as Macmillan nurses, and tend to engender high levels of medicalisation). The therapies on offer in these groups will almost always be of the kind that the biomedical community considers 'safe' (i.e. benign or harmless in their effects on the patient). Similarly, the CAM therapists affiliated to them will generally be subject to intense professional scrutiny, and be subordinate to medical personnel; only those considered to have appropriate credentials, and those willing to abide by this system of accreditation, will be allowed to access patients. In these group environments CAM plays a secondary role – both in relation to biomedical cancer care in general and in relation to the group itself. In this context it effectively becomes just one of a number of discrete activities that group members may choose to be involved in. As such, CAM therapies are not incorporated as part of a wider holistic agenda, and in this way the utilisation of CAM proceeds very much in terms of the biomedical organisational framework (and by extension, the biomedical perspective).

Type 2 groups

These groups, on the other hand, are set up with an overtly holistic agenda. They are generally much smaller in terms of membership, less integrated into wider health networks and underfunded when compared with their NHS-affiliated partners. Their independence allows them to reflect more readily an underlying CAM/holistic ethos because CAM forms an integral part of what they do, and they are generally run and organised by CAM therapists. They still tend to be wary of their image and positioning in relation to biomedicine; however, Type 2 groups tend to encourage a defined and separate 'CAM' identity which Type 1 groups do not usually have. They may display a more liberal attitude towards the qualifications of the therapists they utilise, and similarly, the actual CAMs that are sanctioned may be far more esoteric and 'Category 3' (House of Lords 2000). This is not always the case, however, and at several of our Type 2 case study groups the process of becoming a regular therapist for the group was extremely stringent, reflecting the well established nature of the group and the reputation it wished to maintain.

Originators and organisers

The cornerstones of any support group are the individuals who take part (Damen *et al.* 2000) – the ordinary members, the organisers and facilitators. Much of the analysis of larger structural themes which follows will therefore be grounded in an exploration of the perspectives, motivation and experience of these individuals. Starting a cancer support group, and particularly one that is going to champion CAM, is a particularly challenging process. Individuals who take on what can be a very demanding, and at times, demoralising role, rarely appear to do so as the result of a purely abstract interest in the cancer field. It may be that they have actually had the disease themselves, or that the experience of seeing others going through an emotional and physical trauma stimulates them to act. In the context of CAM, it is often also the case that individuals who have experience of or with a given therapeutic modality – be this reiki healing, special diets, or any number of other CAM approaches – see what they can offer as somehow filling a therapeutic need which is not catered for by current biomedical cancer services. It is common, too, to find (CAM) therapists reporting that the process of engaging with cancer, and confronting it on a professional level, has the incidental effect of stimulating self-development processes that were hitherto unexplored.

> I sat down with myself and thought, there is so much fear around this [cancer] and so much negativity around it that if I can't tackle and face my own fear about it, then I have no business prescribing for people, because, if I'm coming from a fearful place then I am passing that on with my remedy as well and they'll feel it in me – if I can't handle my fear of it then I have no business anywhere near cancer patients. That's my belief. So I sat down and thought, I think I can do this; I think I can release my fear; I think I can look at it as just another disease. Every person who has symptoms or who is ill has a dis-ease with themselves and cancer is just one of many. So I thought, I can put this into perspective – even with people who are suffering from cancer or MS or chronic fatigue or whatever – that they are just an individual out of balance with themselves, and I thought I could do that, and once I thought I could do it, then I started to attract cancer patients, and cancer patients started booking into my clinic. I was put to the test and I found I could do it. I have cancer patients and I can talk to them about the positive side of the illness – that you don't have to accept anyone's prognosis, and the door is always open. As soon as you accept someone's prognosis then the

door is closed. I believe that the body has such a tremendous potential for self-healing although I don't always know how to tap into it or how to advise my patients to tap into it, and I don't always know which way to point them or how to stimulate them, but ultimately the potential for self-healing I think is more tremendous than we imagine.

(Female support group originator and homeopath)

At one level, then, the nature of cancer (i.e. a serious and possibly life-threatening disease) appears to attract a certain kind of CAM therapist, particularly in terms of the pathway which has led them to CAM, and the life narratives that underpin their progress along the route towards an active engagement with cancer care. A number of the therapists and organisers that we interviewed recounted how their connection to a group or to CAM activities in general, was the result of serendipitous or 'guided' coincidence, something which resonates strongly with the spiritual aspects that underpin many CAM modalities. Some such CAM adherents – particularly those of an especially esoteric bent – frequently attributed significance and meaning to what outsiders may consider to be apparently random and coincidental, or indeed planned, events. At one case study group, for example, a therapist repeatedly expressed wonder and surprise at the way in which cancer patients kept 'finding' him. This was in spite of the fact that he operated out of a room in a cancer hospital, had a well established informal referral network and leaflets advertising his services were freely available to patients.

It is common, too, to find other key CAM stakeholders in the group environment (i.e. individuals who are not actually therapists, but who have had direct experience of dealing with cancer patients as a carer to a family member or friend). And as with therapists, it is often the process of first-hand engagement with people who are navigating their way through the trials of biomedical treatment which leads to the development (or entrenchment) of dissatisfaction with aspects of the biomedical approach to cancer care, and their subsequent involvement in support group activities.

There was nothing – this would be about ... around 1980–81, something like that. And looking back I wonder how I coped as much as I did at the time. But, as they say, in those days you just did. There was no alternative. Unfortunately my sister did not survive. But this time [as a result of having cancer myself], I got thoroughly involved in supporting other people. I know Sarah Smith lost her husband round about the same time as I lost my sister. We'd known each other for years. So we then were there to support each other through the loss as well as everything else, and being a very small [support] group you become friends as well as [a source of] support.

(Male support group organiser)

An important dynamic between CAM and cancer is that, as is the case with many other serious illnesses, CAM therapies are rarely the first port of call for patients; even those individuals who have a strong proclivity for CAM are very unlikely to reject biomedicine altogether once they are diagnosed (McGinnis 1990). It is far more common to find CAMs being utilised as a means of mitigating the side effects of chemotherapy or other forms of bio-medical cancer care. Thus, by the time individuals begin exploring the possibility of 'alternatives' they are usually well established on a biomedical treatment regimen. CAM, in this context, can therefore represent a 'last resort' in terms of therapeutic expectations, and this can engender a degree of alienation on the part of therapists. It may, for some therapists, lead to a determination to facilitate 'choice' (i.e. choice to utilise CAM) and support for patients – patients who they may perceive as being locked into a view of health and illness that is needlessly making matters worse for them.

> Because I'd seen cancer patients and I suppose I was amazed at how a lot of them don't think they've got choices. I think a lot of them are frightened and vulnerable. Vulnerable to what people say to them or suggest to them, and it seemed to me that if they are taking on the neg-ative things that people are saying to them – like the fear or 'You must have chemo', then they'd be susceptible to the positive too – like 'You can look at a way of curing yourself'.
>
> (Group originator and CAM therapist)

Group evolution

Despite very real differences within and between group types, it is our con-tention that a recognisable developmental process is observable. Of course, as with the distinction between Type 1 and Type 2 groups, this is not meant to be seen as an inevitable and unfaltering process. But the three phases that we will outline do appear to resonate with the developmental process in our case study groups. It is also consistent, according to the experience of study participants, with the evolution of such groups across the board.

Phase 1: origins

Initially, as a group is beginning to develop there is a burst of enthusiasm. This may originally have been generated as the result of a 'final straw' inci-dent, such as patients being frustrated by a lack of services. Equally, there may have been no negative reasons behind a group's genesis; people may simply have had the desire to provide something that was not currently available. Negative experiences with health professionals were evident in our data, but despite the apparent antipathy between CAM and biomedical practitioners which is often reported, this dynamic was relatively rare.

Phase 1 is characterised by action: people are being approached to become involved and volunteer their services; premises are being found; the first batch of posters advertising the group is being put up, and so on.

> I started talking to people, especially this person, my colleague who I met on a Friday night – you know – a cancer group would be a good idea. People could support themselves and eventually we'd get a bigger group, and you know how you do, you talk about it over coffee and throw it around a bit and as soon as you started talking about it, it changes its energy in that if you are just thinking about it its more like closed energy, but once you throw it out there it nearly takes its own energy. Somebody else heard us talking and they said it would be a good idea and somebody else heard – a good idea as well, and they had lots of questions. Where would you meet? How would you form the group? How would you structure the group and keep it positive? Because what I didn't want it to be like was 'Let's have a cup of tea and a biscuit and my cancer is bigger than your cancer, and my story is worse than your story ...' That wouldn't be a good energy, but how do you not let it become that without coming over as bossy or manipulating or whatever. So I had lots of questions and I thought I had to find the answer to these before I started the group, but then eventually people were talking and people were associating my name, especially in [name of town] with this cancer group thing. So then we went over to meet people from the [name of town] Clinic [support group in neighbouring town] and I actually then challenged myself – do I need answers to these questions? Because there will always be a question, and do we always need to know how to do something? Why not have the courage to take a deep breath and say we are launching this group on 24 June at 1.30 p.m. and it's called cancer support group and see what happens. So I decided to do that.
>
> (Female group originator and CAM therapist)

This initial enthusiasm can last for quite some time, but depending on the aspirations of the organisation (in terms of the kind of contact they seek, or need, from biomedical health networks) it is eventually replaced by a second phase – one often characterised by 'struggle'.

Phase 2: struggle

At this point, even CAM-based groups that are ostensively no threat to biomedicine begin to find the reality of what they are attempting to do and the practicalities of doing it difficult to deal with. For a group organiser entering Phase 2, the initial enthusiasm and potential which characterised the early period of a group's genesis can seem like a naïve dream. This is particularly true of Type 2, or extreme grassroots organisations. Often, the individuals involved in starting these kinds of group are essentially living and breathing the CAM life world; their involvement as therapists or enthusiasts imbues every aspect of their lives, and it may be quite a shock to find that when they attempt to make connections with wider health networks not everyone understands or appreciates their efforts. Even those organisations that follow all the bureaucratic conventions that will make them acceptable to established networks, and are perhaps only offering 'harmless' forms of CAM therapy such as healing or massage, find that it is much more difficult than they imagined to break through into a position where they can operate as an integrated part of the health community. GP surgeries and oncology departments may be reluctant to establish referral networks with a new and unknown group (not necessarily just because they are providing CAM of course, although this will immediately alienate many biomedical health professionals). And even groups that manage to become relatively successful in terms of membership and support can still find fundamental problems with access and engagement in mainstream environments frustrating.

> I think really the connections depend upon the medical profession really. What we have discovered, because we did a little bit of an analysis last quarter, and we've done an awful lot of going round pushing stuff into doctors' surgeries and this, that and the other, and we've said, 'Look, the response from the doctors is not very good. So we are going to concentrate, so far as the GP world is concerned, more upon the nurses'. We thought there is a greater chance of getting a response from the nurses. As far as hospitals are concerned, again it depends on the area. I mean, for example, for many years we did have quite a good connection with [local hospital]. We have various departments that would do things for us, but it depends on the Sister really – who's there. The Breast Care ward in [name of hospital] and [name of hospital] say 'yes, no problem at all', so it depends very much on that. I suppose if you can establish a contact, you can keep it going, and it is often a personal contact that counts.
>
> (Female group organiser, Group 5)

Organisers report finding that it is far more difficult to be 'accepted' and appreciated than they envisaged at the onset of the group. At this point, after perhaps a year or so, a significant number of groups begin to disintegrate. This can happen for a variety of reasons, many of which relate to the practicalities of running any voluntary group: internal politics, originators or key members losing interest, and so on. In the groups that get past this stage, however, organisers and key members can move into a third phase, one characterised by a kind of resigned isolation.

Phase 3: consolidation of identity

Groups that survive into this phase can probably be regarded as 'established'. For Type 1 organisations (which may well have been operating for a long period before offering CAM services) this can be seen as the point at which their provision of CAM is no longer a novelty, and becomes just another part of what they do. For organisers in Type 2 groups, however, Phase 3 is more significant. Having found that parity with biomedically aligned support groups is much more difficult to achieve than they originally imagined, those CAM organisers who are still in the race begin to regard their position as more aligned with that of 'CAM' in a wider sense, something which by definition will always represent a departure from the biomedical system. In a way, they may begin to see themselves as outsiders, but as with many who find themselves in this position, they turn this ostensively negative development to their advantage; they can start to perceive themselves and their group as guardians of perspectives and knowledge that are under threat. Ironically, as we shall explore in more depth in Chapter 6, this position can also benefit an organisation as a whole by drawing members together and strengthening a sense of common identity.

Therapeutic expertise

In the context of disease-specific CAM treatments (as opposed to those that claim general enhancements to wellbeing, and may be utilised by healthy people as well as those who are actually ill), there has, of course, been a history of critical engagement with CAM, its advocates and its practitioners. The notion that 'expertise' is being provided has been a central point of concern. 'Expertise' in a given modality is not a currency which is generally accepted – and certainly not at the same level as medical expertise.

> I had a patient whose breast had gone to cancer, and she said she had sent off to America for some new drug on the internet. She said actually it's – this is what made me sit up – it's from NASA the space agency. It was interesting; it costs I don't know how much, a couple of hundred pounds, and when it came all it was was a hormone that I could have got for £5.60 on prescription from the GP. It was just a hormone that sometimes you use to help appetite as opposed to steroids.
>
> (Male Macmillan nurse)

CAM can be regarded as, at the very least, a naïve distraction, but at worse, something that may be harmful to patients. This is a particularly pertinent discourse in the case of cancer because of the argument that some of the most common CAM-related herbal preparations are actively dangerous when combined with the drugs or processes which form a mainstay of biomedical cancer treatments. St John's wort, a herbal ingredient used by many CAM modalities, is frequently said to be highly reactive when combined with some forms of chemotherapy (Izzo *et al.* 2005; Ernst 2004). Similarly, some topically applied creams and other skin treatments, such as certain oils used in aromatherapy, can, it is argued, have a reactive or screening effect when used in conjunction with radiotherapy (Micke *et al.* 2003).

> ... obviously with some therapies, when you know patients are using certain [CAM] treatments, like massage and things, you are aware that they shouldn't be massaging over certain sites of treatment. Or if there is active disease, you have got to be very careful ... there is a danger they [un-qualified complementary practitioners] may be unaware of the difficulties in the cancer area. I'm not saying they don't mean well, and their heart's in the right place, but what control is there over these practitioners?
>
> (Female Macmillan nurse)

So, in practical terms there are likely to be barriers to group organisers who might be perceived as 'exposing' vulnerable patients to treatments which are outside those sanctioned by the biomedical community. This is one of the reasons why the CAM modalities popular in the majority of support group settings (both Type 1 and Type 2 organisations) are those usually categorised as 'harmless' as far as biomedical practitioners are concerned; hands-on healing, t'ai chi, massage and so on. When practices more contentious are offered (such as homeopathy), confrontation with the gatekeepers who control access to the lifeblood of any support group (i.e. the patients) becomes a possibility.

> ... I think if you want to be taken seriously by the medics and the nurses at this moment in time you have got to stick to the therapies that are tried and tested and are becoming self-regulated as well. This is the big thing with complementary therapies. So I think we started off with aromatherapy and massage which is becoming more and more popular in hospitals as well ... A lot of nurses train to do it. I think it's because they miss the 'hands on' as things become more technical, and maybe the auxiliaries are taking on the caring side of things, which is what I wanted to do when I was nursing. So I think they are going back to it with the complementary therapies.
>
> (Female therapist and group organiser, Group 6)

It can be noted here that some of the more radical and outspoken groups, or more specifically, the key people who run them, can sometimes adopt approaches that underline differences from the mainstream and confirm 'separateness'. Clinics, surgeries, cancer wards and other official (i.e. NHS and medical) environments generally adopt, as part of their public presentations, clear positions that stress how they avoid the sanctioning of anything that could mislead patients, or that might undermine their biomedical treatment (even to the point of displaying publicity material for outside support groups). Having talked to a wide range of CAM therapists about this, it is significant that those who appear to project a more 'conventional' persona (regardless of their underlying beliefs/CAM discipline, etc.) report less 'trouble' in terms of acceptance by key biomedical gatekeepers. It may be, therefore, that the negative or obstructive attitudes which are occasionally reported in relation to biomedical health professionals might originate in misalignments at a micro or interpersonal level, rather than as a consequence of a simple rejection of CAM – a position which several respondents in Type 2 organisations still adhered to despite the apparent shift towards a broader consensus on integration.

While we may identify some CAM group originators, organisers, facilitators and therapists, as CAM 'evangelists' (i.e. individuals who are devoted to publicising a particular kind of treatment or therapy, be it Gerson diets or radionics), in the majority of environments that we investigated, the successful integration of CAM into established support groups, or the inauguration of new groups, depended, to a large extent, on the availability of a wider range of skills – particularly qualities of leadership and organisation. In our data, the contrast between groups that took a 'professional' approach (i.e. in terms of embracing biomedical organisational models) was quite striking; having a veneer of conventionality, and not stressing the polarising aspects of CAM, often worked very well as an integration tool. Looking at the characteristics of these particular CAM-based groups it is evident that they are usually run and maintained by people who, despite having very strong convictions about the efficacy and therapeutic benefit of particular CAM modalities, are able to appreciate that in real terms, integration into the mainstream is still at a relatively early stage and any involvement comes at a price. Often this price is simply being aware of what various key (and sceptical) audiences, such as biomedical health professionals, hospital authorities, and cancer patients themselves, will accept as 'reasonable', and tailoring behaviour accordingly. Successful group organisers – particularly those operating within or near to biomedical settings – soon learn to avoid making claims about their activities that may be considered too far-fetched or esoteric in biomedical terms. They learn, it seems, that even the most open-minded oncologist is unlikely to allow their name to be associated with anything that contains even hints of 'quackery' or 'pseudo-science'. Similarly, others in biomedical healthcare roles have careers to consider, and will be wary of getting labelled as facilitating questionable activities (in biomedical terms).

Successful organisers tend to be disabused of the assumption that people will inevitably and unquestioningly embrace the therapies that they have to offer. And for individuals who can avoid personalising what might be seen as a rejection of their key beliefs, a self-critical adaptation to the position that they find themselves in can be turned to strategic advantage. They learn not to leave themselves open to being perceived as a threat – either to the credibility of the local health networks they seek to engage with, or to the existing authority of biomedical clinicians. They understand notions of 'evidence' and 'efficacy' as espoused by biomedical clinicians, and position themselves and their activities as supplementary (and by implication, subordinate) to biomedicine. They will, for example, emphasise that the meditation sessions they are offering are very similar to 'relaxation' and there will be no mention of auras, angels or the ethereal body.

A final issue which appears to motivate people to organise and run support groups with a significant CAM element is the perception that the apparent demand for CAM-based services is not being met by current health provision. Although there has been a growth of interest in CAM by cancer sufferers, the actual availability of therapies (particularly in terms of the NHS) is still very patchy. Despite health policies which have begun to actively encourage an element of integration (DoH 2001; Calman and Hine 1995), there is currently no overall plan for its implementation and consequently little real funding for initiatives. The high-profile activities of organisations dedicated to encouraging integration between CAM and biomedicine, such as the Prince of Wales's Foundation for Integrated Health,[2] have played their part in raising expectations about the availability of CAM services (Pinder *et al.* 2005). Similarly, in particular relation to cancer, well established charities such as Macmillan Cancer Relief have helped build the credibility of certain modalities by producing directories of therapies for cancer patients, and information on where support groups that offer them are located (Kohn 1999). What this ascendant profile has meant, however, is that although cancer patients' expectations about the usefulness of CAM can be high, in practical terms much CAM is available only privately, and is therefore still beyond the means of many people. Despite all of the sociopolitical motivations which have frequently been seen to underpin a large proportion of the CAM world – ranging from ecological awareness through to spirituality – the majority of practitioners do not routinely provide their services for free.[3] The actual cost of consulting, say, a homeopath or acupuncturist, can be relatively high. This is particularly true when treatments require ongoing or multiple consultations – a situation which is likely to arise with conditions such as cancer. Even cancer care 'standards' such as hands-on healing or reflexology can be expensive if paid for on a one-to-one basis.

The discrepancy between the perceived good that CAM can do for patients, and patients' ability to access CAM services, can therefore become a significant driving factor behind the formation of groups. In several of our Type 2/grassroots organisations, for example, this was a key motivational factor. From our observations we found that often organisers who are themselves CAM therapists will utilise the voluntary and altruistic nature of the support group environment to encourage other practitioners to offer their services to members at either a greatly reduced rate, or free of charge. Similarly, groups that are CAM focused, but which do not necessarily have access to therapists as key members, can utilise their openness to holistic ideals to attract practitioners who might wish to give demonstrations or short sample sessions (either to the group as a whole, or on a one-to-one basis). This system works to the mutual benefit of both parties: the group members are able to take advantage of CAMs that they might not otherwise have been able to access, and the therapists who provide these sessions are able to feel that they are contributing to the wellbeing and success of the group (and by extension, the wider community). Raising awareness of their particular therapeutic modality (and CAM/holism in general) is also a useful by-product of the arrangement, as is the follow-up business that group members have the potential to generate for these practitioners.

Most of our case study groups utilised this type of arrangement, usually with one or more of the main stakeholders providing a 'key' therapy for which the group became known (natural healing, for example, in Group 1; dietary nutrition and lifestyle advice in Group 2, and movement therapies in Group 8). These base activities would then be augmented by other therapies as and when practitioners were willing to provide them. A slight variation on this system was operated in Group 5. Here, the main function of the twice monthly group meetings was for stakeholders to explore, and try out for free, an eclectic range of therapies.

When deciding which therapies (and therapists) to involve, organisers reported being very conscious that the forum they were offering could be open to people with less than altruistic motivations.

> What we tend to do is when somebody [a CAM therapist] shows an interest, we invite them to join us on a non-functioning basis, just to see what happens for at least a couple of occasions to see if they want to join or if we feel they are suitable. I can only remember one time when we had a little bit of doubt about somebody – although he was qualified, he didn't seem ... so we tactfully discouraged him from coming again. But normally it's the other way around; people are trying to find out if they wish to do something on a voluntary basis when they would probably be getting paid for their services outside. One thing we insist on is that they don't self-advertise with us. We don't want them to do that for obvious reasons.
>
> (Group organiser, Group 5)

Patient engagement with CAM

We now turn to a brief overview of some significant features of patient engagement with CAM in support groups. It is important to bear in mind that discussions here relate specifically to use of therapies in this organisational context. A broader range of issues dealing with individual engagement with the plurality of therapeutic options will be considered in much greater depth elsewhere (Broom and Tovey, forthcoming).

The way in which cancer patients, and the plethora of other stakeholders they engage with as they deal with their illness, conceptualise CAM can obviously be a significant factor in determining how, when, and if they decide to engage with the kinds of support groups that offer CAM services. From our data, it is evident that there really is no one particular type of person, particular kind of outlook, set of beliefs or perspective that characterises the individuals who decide to utilise CAM in their cancer care. Nor is it possible to predict who will find that CAM is commensurable with their personal view of health and illness. Similarly, there seems to be no way of knowing who will be likely to reject it, and at what point in the illness trajectory they may do this. At an organisational level, the only significant commonality appears to be that virtually everyone involved in this field has either had first-hand experience of cancer, or has nursed, cared for or supported a relative or friend with the disease.

> My wife and I both have cancer, and I was in at the beginning [of the support group]. The woman who founded the centre, she had a very close friend who died of cancer, and they were both conscious of the lack of simple support in the medical profession. They didn't blame anybody for that – it's just a fact it wasn't there. So I think that's how it began and it's 13 years old now. When it began, and from that quite tentative beginning we've got a lot more people ... so I think it sustains itself fairly well, not to say we don't go through anxiety, but fairly well.
> (Male group originator, Group 5)

In terms of the types of patient who access CAM in the group environments we are concerned with, again, there appear to be no particularly idiosyncratic qualities by which they can be singled out. Admittedly, there is a significant gender bias evident across the broad range of cancer support groups; women routinely outnumber men by quite a large margin, but even taking this into account (and the usage studies which have largely categorised the average CAM user as white, middle-class and female (e.g. Thomas *et al.* 2001), a myriad of different perspectives on healthcare, cancer and CAM are evident. This in many ways reflects the eclectic appropriation of CAM in wider society (in the sense that multiple modalities are routinely incorporated by users).

Rationale for involvement with CAM can be very straightforward. The primary reason that many patients may initially engage with the CAM therapies that support groups offer may simply be a desire to try anything that will help them deal with their cancer and/or alleviate biomedical treatment side effects. While many hold a strong belief in the efficacy of CAM(s), it seems that for most patients the CAM they access through support groups is just another avenue to be pursued in the hope that life can be prolonged, or quality of life maintained.

> ... [the session] was nothing mind-shattering, you know; no road to Damascus thing, it was pleasant and I went away; I did go away feeling a bit better and also while I was in [the healing group] the nurse that had told me to go had actually come out of the clinic and brought me a little book, *Bad Hair Days*, it was an American publication written for women with cancer and had lost their hair, and it was kind of one-liners, and she had actually gone to the trouble to leave a busy clinic and she said, 'Here, I thought you might like this; it will make you smile', and it did, and I thought how nice it was to go to that trouble, and I went away and I felt a little better.
>
> (Female, 44 years, lung cancer)

CAM in the context of cancer support is often less encumbered by the esoteric contextualisations which may infuse CAM use in other settings. This may be partly because the medical specialism with which it must engage (i.e. oncology) is very much disease focused and places little emphasis on emotional or spiritual aspects of the treatment process. Cancer treatments are routinely at the cutting edge of medical science, while certain CAM modalities often make a virtue of looking back and re-assimilating 'old' or 'lost' therapeutic knowledge; CAM therapists usually place an emphasis on the holistic and non-invasive nature of what they do, while biomedical cancer treatments routinely have harsh side effects, focusing on the physiological elements of disease.

The largely pragmatic approach to CAM so often found amongst cancer patients may also have a lot to do with the nature of the disease. Even when the prognosis is good, cancer is perceived as a life-threatening illness, and brings with it a raft of psychological implications. What is particularly striking about many of the patients who utilise CAM as part of the support group process – particularly those who find themselves facing the possibility of imminent death, or the onset of severe pain – is the shift which can occur in their beliefs about, and relationship to, the CAM therapies they are involved in. Although CAM is often portrayed as synonymous with self-development, holism and spirituality, it seems that for many people with serious pain or terminal illness, the relevance of these qualities can (initially at least) be quickly subsumed. When matters of pure survival become significantly more pressing, the 'fashionable' aspects of CAM use as 'lifestyle', which delineate it as a singularly late-modern consumer phenomenon, are subsumed by more critical and physiologically focused conceptions of treatment validity. Those that are of no practical benefit (in terms of tangible results right now) are quickly dropped.

> ... I ask, 'Will this help cure me?' If not, I'm not going to waste time on it. I don't have time for bullshit; I literally don't have time ...
>
> (Male, 47 years, lung cancer)

The rejection of esoteric and spiritual elements within CAM is by no means universal though, and in some cases interesting re-emergent dynamics come into play as people become socialised into a 'CAM' mindset. This tends to be either as a result of contact with a group or as a result of personal explorations as they find that a particular CAM ethos resonates with them.

> ... some patients don't come back. It's often because it's not what they want to hear; they want someone to do it for them. And I think possibly the way I practise is that I encourage my patients to take responsibility for their own healing and right from day one.
>
> (Female, CAM therapist/group organiser, Group 1)

Whether or not the wider holistic/self-empowerment subtext of CAM is sidelined in favour of pure therapeutic efficacy, it seems that it remains available – even to those who initially reject it. The nature of CAM routinely encourages patients to engage simultaneously with psychological, social and spiritual issues which may go well beyond the purely medical and overtly symptomatic. Take the example of the natural (or 'spiritual' healing) which is such a mainstay of CAM provision in cancer care: it is possible to engage with this modality in a completely secular way – to treat a 'hands-on' session or group work as a purely physical therapy. However, even a limited experience of the process (and one in which the therapist actively avoids offering any esoteric explanations for what is occurring) is likely to stimulate curiosity about what exactly it is that is 'going on' – how the often dramatic relief from stress and worry, and the multiplicity of visual and physical effects so often reported by patients undergoing healing, is actually achieved.

For some people, exposure to, and engagement with, CAM has the effect of stimulating intense periods of self-reflection and self-development. Our data is littered with accounts of patients who reported being in some way more 'open' to the therapeutic possibilities of self-empowerment (in terms of control over a part of their treatment process) that occurred once they took a serious interest in some form of CAM. Although it is, of course, difficult to ascertain whether these new-found attitudes are due to exposure to the CAM processes themselves, or to the significant mental adaptations that dealing with the stress of a potentially terminal illness can engender. Many people find reserves of strength and resolve that they had previously been unaware of when faced with extreme situations.

Contact with CAM in the support/self-help group context (which is by implication, part of the process of self-empowerment) can similarly be an important means by which people who would not ordinarily have any interest in the field can become a locus of propagation. Enthusiastic group members will play an important role in leading their fellow patients towards CAM. Being cancer patients themselves, they have a built-in level of credibility which therapists and 'lay' members may not have no matter how empathetic they may try to be. This credibility is further enhanced if the therapy or process under recommendation appears to be effective.

Significantly, although practical issues such as the unpleasant and damaging side effects of biomedical treatments do crop up, the reservations that many stakeholders have with biomedicine do not necessarily relate to its efficacy per se. More often cited are concerns about the shortcomings of its delivery and the provision of aftercare. Cancer patients can be reticent about the routinely debilitating side effects of chemotherapy, for example, because they may perceive it as something necessary which simply has to be endured in order to effect a cure; it is, after all, the 'best' that biomedicine can offer and the 'best' way to beat the cancer. What is clear, however, both in data generated as a result of this project, and much of the literature concerning the subjective experience of patients (e.g. Furnham 1996; Montbriand 1998), is that many patients are concerned about the increasing technologicalisation and depersonalisation of biomedical cancer care. Not only may treatments have unpleasant and debilitating side effects, but their actual application (i.e. often via complex machines, and with the patient in isolated or uncomfortable environments) may be equally disturbing.

In this chapter we have begun to focus on some of the broad structural issues which underpin the development and organisation of CAM-based cancer support groups. A key element of our analysis has been the idea that most organisations fall into one of two categories: those that were well established as support groups before beginning to provide CAM services, and those that were set up with an overtly CAM/holistic agenda. Through an exploration of the reasoning and motivation which characterises the individuals who organise and take part in these main types of support group, we have described the ongoing and unavoidable influence that paradigmatic tensions between biomedicine and CAM have on the way in which groups develop and function. In the next chapter we will begin to narrow our focus and examine the way in which key activities such as information utilisation and decision making on CAM are enacted by stakeholders as they engage in support group activities.

Chapter 4

Group performance

Enacting therapeutic alternatives in the collective environment

The mediation of CAM in and by support groups can be analysed at two distinct, but fundamentally interdependent, levels: on a macro level, patient support organisations can be said to be at the forefront of CAM provision – they appear to be, after all, a key nexus between the world of CAM and the world of the patient. However, this is only a small part of the picture. Cancer care may well be at the cutting edge of integration, but it must be remembered that only a relatively small number of disparate therapies are routinely offered to cancer patients (that is, in the context of contact through support groups) (Kohn 1999). Moreover, as we shall see, the therapeutic landscapes that these limited therapies engender are often not representative of CAM in its myriad forms.

Aside, then, from the broader position that patient support groups occupy within healthcare structures, community networks and society as a whole, it is important that analysis at a micro-interactional – or at least an interactional level – is incorporated into an approach geared towards enhancing understanding of the area. Given that this whole field is still relatively under-researched (Chatwin and Tovey 2004), the question of what actually goes on between interactants (i.e. group members, group organisers, CAM therapists, biomedical health workers and so on) when they engage in CAM-related activities is highly salient.

This chapter will be based around an exploration of the activities that occurred during a routine meeting at one of our case study groups (Group 1). Basing our discussion on an in-depth case study will enable us to give a detailed description of a discrete 'CAM' environment (something which will be useful for readers unfamiliar with the conventions of the area). We selected the group in question because it provides an interesting insight into the functioning of support groups. Of course, it has its own very specific history, organisation and group processes. And, as such, caution should be used in using this as a 'representative' example of all such groups. Having said this, the kinds of structures observed in this group and the kinds of issues that arose did have a resonance across all the fieldwork sites. It is evident, for instance, that the operationalisation of CAM therapies themselves

– the way in which they were performed – had noticeable similarities across groups. They had, as such, easily recognisable formats. The experience of a guided meditation session, for example, was much the same wherever it took place. And the same could be said of t'ai chi or an aromatherapy massage session. Essentially, then, the case study that follows, while not intended as a definitive illustration of 'the way things are' across the board, does provide a means of accessing the way in which CAM processes are enacted in CAM/cancer support groups beyond the individual case cited.

Central to our analysis here will be the structural and interactional elements of groups, and in particular, the interrelation between the two. We will explore how the activities and approach of groups are unavoidably related to the expertise and background of key organisers, a dynamic which can create tension on several levels. Similarly, we will examine the tensions which arise between the location and enactment of CAM processes, and explore whether or not differences in the aims and objectives of cancer support groups (as opposed to recreational CAM or 'lifestyle' focused groups) might affect factors such as membership and membership turnover. Does the 'open access' format (i.e. where carers and non-patients are actively encouraged to participate in activities) have a significant impact on the way group sessions are run? Does the accommodation of new and 'CAM-inexperienced' members alongside individuals with much greater CAM-related knowledge impact on group processes? A common feature of many CAM modalities found in the cancer support group setting is the formal or informal 'debriefing' which follows the completion of group sessions. Does the experiential knowledge exchange that this represents have a varying emphasis and role in different group settings? We will also deal with issues arising from the ways in which stakeholders interpret and utilise information on CAM – how therapists and organisers overcome the conflict between biomedical and CAM paradigms which forms an unavoidable backdrop to what they do.

The case study

> Sometimes when you think there's no way out of a situation, that situation is taken out of your hands. I was in a situation and I found things that I would never have found. For one thing I wouldn't have found meditation; I most definitely would not. And I just think, well, now that I've found it I'm going to hold onto it. 'Cos every time I meditated, I felt so much better. When I looked round at the other patients who were going through exactly the same as me, I couldn't believe how well I felt, and how I just seemed to sail through it. Even the consultant couldn't believe it at times because the side effects that you're supposed to have with this really strong chemo[therapy] – I just didn't get any.
>
> (Female, 50 years, Group 3, breast cancer)

This case study will focus on a single meeting of Group 3. This group is unusual because it does not readily conform to a Type 1 or Type 2 categorisation. In fact, it probably fits somewhere between the two, retaining certain key characteristics of both. This makes it a useful place from which to begin illustrating the workings of a CAM-focused support group because the ambiguities which underlie its position incorporate a number of interactional dynamics that are routinely exclusive to 'pure' groups from the extremes of the continuum. Its hybrid nature also means, of course, that it has distinct and idiosyncratic qualities that are not normally evident in these organisations.

Support group location

Although physically based in a cancer hospital for the last eighteen years or so, Group 3 is actually relatively isolated, particularly in terms of connections to wider healthcare networks and, surprisingly, within its host institution. Its activities are not widely known about, even among the staff working on the wards from which it draws the majority of its members. There are similarly no formal systems in place whereby healthcare staff at the hospital can refer patients, and it is largely through informal contacts and the individual efforts of the group organiser that patients find out about the CAM activities that are available to them.

The group was started and is currently still run by a single CAM therapist. This particular therapist classifies herself as a 'natural' healer, and is keen not to be labelled a 'spiritual' healer. This reflects her desire to play down any esoteric or metaphysical associations that this label might generate for patients (and hospital staff) – a situation that crops up quite often in groups that in any way rely on biomedical networks. This also meant that any crossover with the 'services' offered by the chaplain was avoided. This therapist takes on all of the tasks involved with the day-to-day organisation of the support group. These include arranging the weekly meetings, designing and delivering the relaxation and meditation exercises which are their focus and keeping informal records of group membership, etc. Significantly, it is this single therapist who provides all of the CAM services to the group, and who is almost exclusively seen as its key member. Only on very rare occasions are other therapists invited to provide activities for group sessions. In fact, during the year or so in which we conducted fieldwork with the group, this occurred only once, and was due to the main therapist being ill.

Unlike most other organisations of this size and type (both Type 1 and Type 2), the CAM therapy ('natural healing') that is the focus for the group meetings is inextricably linked to the personal talents and reputation of the main organiser. She is, for example, a widely known and well established CAM healer in her own right and has a very strong personal reputation with cancer patients in the local region.[4] This reputation, however – in a dynamic which is common in other groups that attempt to cross over into the territory of biomedical service provision – appears to make little difference when it comes to the practicalities of integration. A reoccurring theme reported by this therapist was the difficulty that she encountered in forming collegial (i.e. equal) relationships with biomedical health professionals (particularly senior oncologists). While, as we have argued already, this kind of difficulty is relatively common for the more independent CAM groups, it is particularly significant that it was such an issue for this organisation, situated as it was in the heart of a cancer hospital, and operating with the support of hospital funding. It is noteworthy that, despite the high degree of official 'legitimisation' which these factors might routinely convey, the therapist (as a CAM practitioner, and one practising what some might view as a particularly 'soft' modality) still felt largely excluded from the primarily biomedical environment in which she operated. Similarly, her position was not helped by the fact that her employment status at the hospital was fundamentally ambiguous. Rather than there being recognisable management and organisational structures within which she could locate herself, she essentially relied to a large degree on the good will and patronage of significant gatekeepers such as specific senior consultants. Several of these key individuals within the hospital understood and valued what she did (coupled, of course, with a significant number of others who did not). Understandably, this tenuous support – valuable though it was – did not necessarily translate into useful and broad working relationships on a day-to-day basis.

The therapist's consulting room was not big enough for more than three or four people to use at any one time, so this required that group meetings be held in an adjacent communal area (see Figure 4.1). This arrangement was not ideal given that the consulting rooms and offices of various other healthcare staff and administrators were also situated around this area. This made through traffic and noise a constant issue during group sessions (which required a quiet and undisturbed environment): sessions were regularly plagued by telephones ringing in nearby offices, doors banging and the generally unavoidable background noise of activity.[5] Even notices pinned to the door asking for quiet during sessions were seemingly ignored, and it was evident that relations between the therapist and other staff who utilised the communal area could be strained in this respect. Despite her efforts to integrate (by, for example, inviting the occupants of the offices to take part in sessions) and make her use of the space as non-disruptive as possible, the activities of the group appeared to be tolerated rather than embraced. This may have simply been connected to a non-appreciation of just how distracting ambient noise can be when people are trying to meditate, rather than anything overtly antagonistic. However, difficulties such as this cropped up again and again in connection with the group to the point where the main therapist now perceived herself to be something of an outsider within the hospital, and had resigned herself to having to struggle to maintain her position and have the value of her activities acknowledged.

> ... the consultants may just regard this [natural healing] as something that is happening, or they may just be putting up with it. Some of them of course have been very supportive – amazingly supportive, and refer patients to me direct. The nurses certainly will pick up the phone and phone me at home if they can see anybody who's in the least little bit struggling. But, how to explain this [healing therapy] to staff who are engrossed in the material and medical world is very difficult. I feel accepted more now – not by everybody, I never would be accepted by everybody, and this isn't for everybody – but there has to be a menu, there has to be choice. So we've got an à la carte menu and we pick out what we feel is for us, and if it's not, fair enough.
>
> (Group leader, CAM therapist, Group 3)

The therapeutic activities of the group organiser were fundamentally tied to the activities of the support group. Her main function within the hospital (and the one for which the hospital paid) was to offer one-to-one hands-on healing and relaxation therapy services to patients. These she usually performed in her consulting room, but she also regularly toured the wards to attend to patients who had requested to see her, or who were too ill to be taken to her room.

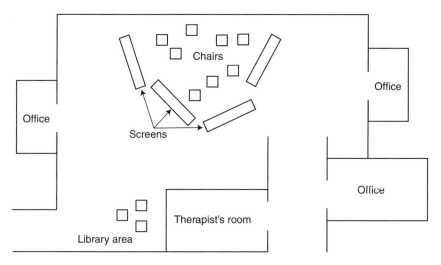

Figure 4.1 Layout of the group area

For anybody who has no awareness at all of what this is about, a natural healing session has nothing to do with religion or beliefs, it's
about letting go – just learning to let go – just being – just feeling safe.
This is not hypnosis or hypnotherapy; this is just saying, look, let's
clear the mind, let's try and empty the mind. Let's try and go past
everything that we think we know, into a void, into a nothingness.
And then out of the nothingness, out of the stillness, then all this
[healing] can come spontaneously ...

(Group leader, CAM therapist, Group 3)

Although an accredited member of the Association of Spiritual Healers, the
strand of healing therapy that she had developed was fairly unusual in the
context of the NHS environment in which she worked (in the sense that even
in CAM terms it was non-standard, being largely based on the idiosyncratic
meditative qualities of her voice, rather than the 'laying on' of hands). This,
however, made her approach particularly suitable for group work in a way
that more 'standard' and wholly tactile approaches may not have been.
Healing practices – particularly those based on prayer or religious beliefs –
are often performed in large groups, but this can be a limitation, allowing the
'hands-on' practitioner only a few minutes with any given participant. It was
an awareness of the potential that her spoken technique had for reaching
larger numbers of people that led her to develop group sessions.[6] She also
reported appreciating that while many patients found the one-to-one experience very powerful, for others, the dynamics of a group setting (including, of
course, the attendant social dimension of sharing the therapeutic experience)
were more appealing. The format of the group, however, was grounded
directly in its practical meditation and relaxation activities, and the purpose
of the weekly meetings was simply to perform these. Meetings were not
overtly structured to incorporate the other elements which are normally
found in support group settings. In particular, 'formal' time for patients to
talk about issues that concerned them was offered after sessions, but it did
not form a key part of the therapeutic process.

Meetings

Routinely, the support group would meet once a week at the hospital.
These sessions were augmented by a regular weekend meeting which took
place in a local hotel. Although following a very similar format (i.e. basically guided group meditations), and open to the same selection of cancer
patients and other stakeholders who attended the hospital, the 'sister'
group tended to attract larger numbers of participants – often 20 or more.
Similarly, the make-up of participants tended to represent more strongly
carers and cancer patients who were either in remission or clear of cancer,
the non-medical environment apparently being more appealing to them.

There was a significant degree of crossover however, with some individuals attending both groups on a regular basis. It was noticeable that patients and carers who were newly introduced to the healing therapy offered at one or other of the groups (and via one-to-one sessions with the therapist), and who found it to be beneficial, tended to go through a period of intense participation, attending as many sessions as they could. This dynamic could be observed at most of our groups, regardless of the CAM modalities on offer.

For the purposes of this case study, we will concentrate on a meeting held at the hospital-based group, as this forms a relatively self-contained environment. During the course of our fieldwork, the number of people attending varied from six to 14, although as many as 24 are reported to have taken part on occasion. Exactly how many individuals would appear in any given week, and the mix of patients, carers, or members of staff, is difficult to predict. Although there were a few 'core' individuals who had been attending both this and the hotel group for many years (and one in particular who had been coming since their inception), turnover of members was relatively high.[7] There were a number of reasons for this. The main one was probably that many cancer sufferers attending the hospital group were more likely to be seriously ill and often died from their illness. A second and equally important factor, however, was that the people who recovered often no longer saw the group as relevant to them. It was perceived as an element of the treatment process, helping them deal with the process of being treated, rather than as a generally life-enhancing activity. This is an area where the dynamics of participation in CAM activities via a support group may be clearly differentiated from those of, say, a recreational meditation group. Although the actual CAM processes observed in recreational groups (i.e. the act of group meditation, etc.) may be indistinguishable from those utilised in a support group environment, participants in recreational groups do not necessarily have any objective other than participation for its own sake, and are unlikely to have any particular illness or problem in common. This means that membership and attendance turnover will rarely be as high as in a group where essentially individualistic goals (i.e. remission, anxiety and stress relief, etc.) are paramount.

Similarly, as we explored in Chapter 3, even though patients in remission or clear of cancer were actively encouraged to continue being part of the group, they very often felt that the associations engendered by the hospital environment were something they no longer wished to engage with. This could be for very pragmatic reasons: in order to attend, patients had to walk past the wards and theatres where they had been treated, and this understandably triggered stressful associations they were not keen to relive. This situation was commonly reported in relation to other groups that operated in similarly 'medical' environments. In the Australian case study group dealt with in Chapter 6, for example, the room utilised for meetings was likewise located right in the heart of a cancer hospital, making it a difficult place to return to for people who did not wish to be reminded of unpleasant treatment experiences.

An interesting variation on this dynamic was the way in which carers of members that had recently died often continued to attend the group and take part in activities for some time afterwards. Again, this behaviour could be observed at several other groups, and was often actively encouraged by organisers. Non patient, carer members at this group would also sometimes be found taking one-to-one healing sessions with the therapist, even if they had not done so during their prior contact with her or the group. It was also interesting to observe that people in this position often felt that they would like to make some sort of positive contribution to the future of the group or, more specifically, to the therapist who embodied it. As direct monetary donations were not considered appropriate (given that services were not being provided on a purely charitable basis), help frequently took the form of practical donations of equipment or services. One relative of a patient, for example, provided a water cooler for the consultation room after the hospital refused to supply one. Another offered printed stationery, and another provided bookshelves for the library.

The therapist's room similarly brimmed with crystals, pictures, candles and ornaments which had been given by grateful patients and their carers, and even the hotel room where the weekend meetings were held was provided free by an ex-patient (the hotel owner) who had been a regular group member when he was treated at the hospital. Other groups in our cohort had a similar reliance on 'payment-in-kind' arrangements, particularly in terms of volunteers to help with stewarding large group meetings where multiple activities might be offered. Group 5 was a particularly good example of this, and could not have functioned without the freely given help of non-members. To some extent, the nature of the cancer support group arena lends itself to these types of arrangements very well, and there are several empirical examples of groups obtaining far more 'good will' from landlords and administrators than might be afforded organisations with less altruistic motivations.

Reciprocation

Apart from showing their appreciation for the help and support that had been provided, the often extremely generous behaviour of individuals towards groups can possibly be explained in terms of the way in which CAM therapies can be perceived to be a help to those bearing the stress of caring for cancer patients, and not just the patients themselves. In our case study group, it is also clear that apart from the actual services that she offered, the therapist was widely considered to be an intuitive and caring person with an in-depth understanding of the perspectives of both patients and carers. This clearly had an effect in the sense that it generated a degree of loyalty amongst those who felt she had helped them or the person they cared for. As is common with many key stakeholders who become involved, either with starting, or running cancer support groups (see Chapter 3), she had herself lost a close relative to cancer, and although she rarely mentioned this directly, it appears to have given her a definite edge when it came to quickly establishing trust and empathy with cancer sufferers.

This experiential legitimacy underlies the open membership approach of many cancer support groups; few, if any, limit their membership to only those who are ill. Certainly this was the case with the groups we worked with. Apart from, that is, those groups that were purely treatment based, and even these tended to have carer support networks in place on top of their other services. It can be said that this actively inclusive approach makes CAM therapies and the kinds of other activities that they engender particularly attractive. Relaxation or meditation can be practised by everyone, not just those who are ill, and this is true of a whole range of CAM modalities, even those that are much more illness focused. This inclusion of all members in a common activity can serve not only as a means of strengthening a group (in terms of shared experiences, etc.), but can also help to lessen the experiential distance between those who are ill and those who are not.

First-timers

For the high proportion of patients who are completely new to the idea of meditation, or knew little of what to expect from a 'CAM' group experience, the first time they take part in a group session can understandably be a little strange. Even though in CAM terms what actually occurs is usually relatively straightforward and carries little of the esoteric character that can underline a sense of difference in CAM-related activities, events usually need to be carefully orchestrated to be as 'natural' as possible (in the sense that meditation, say, is presented as an activity in which participants simply access a natural human ability, and are not required to buy into any particular religious or spiritual belief system). This is particularly important in environments where completely new members are encouraged to 'drop in' – a situation which is largely universal in these types of support organisations. To this end, the therapist in our present case study would usually try to meet participants as they arrived. Routinely, as members entered the main group area (see Figure 4.1), those familiar with the workings of the group would gather in and around the small library area. The therapist would also try to stay in this area so that she was available to talk to any new arrivals, explain what was going to occur, and head off anyone who might be potentially disruptive, or who might not find the group to their taste. Surprisingly, this could be a significant problem – people with strong religious beliefs were reportedly particularly troublesome, but the objective here was definitely not to exclude; rather it was to ensure that the meeting went smoothly and nothing that occurred was offensive to anyone's sensibilities. Gradually, as it came nearer to the time when the session was due to start, people would move towards the circle of chairs.

Figure 4.1 illustrates the layout of the communal area where the group sessions took place. Before people were due to arrive, the therapist would position ten or so chairs in a circle towards one end of the room and pull hospital screens around it to give a degree of privacy. However, as we have already outlined, this did nothing to exclude the noise from nearby offices. Often, a small table was positioned in the centre of the circle on which were placed a selection of large quartz crystals. The displaying of crystals in such a prominent position is significant because objects of this type can be said to be unambiguous symbols of the more esoteric aspects of CAM: they tend to be a ubiquitous presence in environments where CAM therapies are provided, often simply as decorative additions, or, as in the case of questionable Category 3 therapies (House of Lords 2000) such as 'crystal healing', as therapeutic tools in their own right. In most other group settings that we were able to observe (particularly Type 1), the display of such objects was largely avoided because they tended to shift the atmosphere of the group too far towards the esoteric – something which usually needed to be underplayed in overtly medical environments if the credibility of the CAM activities was not to be stretched too far. In this group, however, the use of (often extremely impressive) crystals as therapeutic props was not curtailed, and on occasion they were even passed around among members – some of whom enthusiastically embraced them as totems of healing power.

Once all the participants were seated, the therapist began her routine. We observed this process on many occasions, and the transcript that follows is representative of a typical session. Being very experienced at performing this type of group meditation, the therapist utilised no notes or prompts. In order to signal that the session was about to begin, she pulled closed the screens which surrounded the chair circle, and turned on a DVD player.[8] On this occasion, soft classical music was used. She then took her seat and spoke to the group.

> Well, welcome everybody. This is the [group name] cancer support group where we do relaxation and hands-on healing. The group's been together for many years and we feel like a very big family. So if some of you are new to this, and you'd like to join in with the session today, what we do is first of all, is to just relax, get comfortable in our chairs, settle down and close our eyes ... Now, just focusing on our breathing ...

> ... Just using our breathing to carry us into an altered state of awareness that's just a very, very deep state of relaxation ...

... and we travel what seems to be, beyond the everyday world with our problems and difficulties, to another state of being – almost like another world that we're tapping into, that runs alongside the everyday world, and most people don't even know it exists, or may go through life totally unaware of it ...

... but it takes a trauma, and a challenge in our lives to make us start thinking, and perhaps find something like this that will help us through ... whatever difficulty presents itself to us in outer life. Whether it be bereavement, illness – any life process that brings any form of crisis ...

... and so it teaches us to let go of it and find something else from within ourselves that we can draw through to help us. Something which isn't a drug ... it isn't toxic ... and it has no side effects. It's finding another part of ourselves ...

... so together, we attune as one. Forgetting momentarily our outer lives, and stress ... and difficulties. We become ... just who we are, on this deeper level ... and what we are doing is addressing our spirituality ... another part of ourselves. Call it the life force ... it's a state of being that brings into our outer lives a feeling of peace, of serenity and calm ... Allowing us to alter those sleep patterns that have kept us asleep every night ... to cope with the situations that present ... to bring energy where it's been depleted ... and helping us to rise above the situation we find ourselves in ... with a sense of calm and dignity ...

At this point, the music was allowed to play on as the therapist walked around behind the group. All participants were now apparently in a very deep state of relaxation with their eyes closed. She paused behind each person for a minute or so and performed a variation of a short 'hands-on' treatment: making several passes over them, then resting her hands, palms down, lightly on their shoulders. Once she had visited every person, she sat back down and allowed the music to play for a further ten minutes or so. The therapist then proceeded to close the meditation.

Okay ... come back everybody ... slowly, in your own time ... make sure you feel grounded, and you're back in this world – if you travelled to another one. Just open your eyes, and come back to the everyday world ... bringing with you strength, confidence and the ability to sleep well ... which all comes from within yourself.

For the next few minutes the group gradually 'came round', opening their eyes and stretching their legs. There was very little conversation, water was passed around in paper cups, and people remained in their seats. Gradually, people began to talk quietly and the therapist brought the focus back on her by asking the group as a whole how they had found the session.

The initiation of an evaluation sequence at this point is significant because regardless of the specific CAM therapy or process being enacted, group sessions such as this will virtually always incorporate some kind of post-completion feedback or activity-related discussion. The way in which this is conducted can vary from formalised procedures in which participants are asked in turn to describe the experience they have just had, through to informal and relatively loose arrangements which overtly address the fact that not everyone will find the process of talking particularly appealing – especially, as in this case, after emerging from what may have been a deep meditative state.

In this group, attention was focused very much on the healing therapy itself, rather than the sharing of subjective experiences relating to it. While the therapist acknowledged the usefulness of groups which encouraged 'talk' as a form of therapeutic exercise in its own right (as in many of the more 'conventional' support group environments), she was keen that her group was not seen as overtly engendering this kind of activity – that is, the emphasis was on the active process of actually *doing* meditation and relax-ation, rather than trying to make sense of what it was or how it worked. The way in which the therapist approached the issue of post-session feed-back was usually just to make a few comments relating to how she herself had found the group that day – perhaps mentioning how she had felt it was a 'strong' or 'deep' session. The emphasis here would be on the collective quality of the experience, rather than any individual person's apparent part in it. This served to concretise the dynamics of the group experience and define it as something distinct from (and often more powerful than) any-thing an individual might achieve on their own.

If there were new participants in the group, the therapist would usually enquire at this point how they had found their first session, and then let anyone else who wished to comment, or ask questions, have the floor. In this particular group setting, these post-therapy discussions rarely went on for any length of time and were not animated affairs. This may well have been due to the intensive relaxation effect that the therapy seemed to have had on people.[9] There were other reasons, too, why she preferred not to encourage too much in-depth analysis among members at this point. These related quite directly to issues of group cohesion. Although this particular session example can be said to have proceeded smoothly, things are not always so straightforward. The therapist reported that leaving the group completely open to anyone inevitably meant that sometimes it would attract people who had strong views (for or against CAM, for example) or those who found the methods she utilised problematic on religious grounds. During fieldwork, for example, one particular individual joined a session (which, like the present example, involved participants closing their eyes and relaxing) and then spent the entire time staring menacingly at the therapist. It later emerged that the person had strong religious beliefs and had been told by a priest that meditation involved 'letting in the Devil'. Why she had come to the group in the first place was not clear, but her presence effectively disrupted activities. She left without comment as soon as the meditation was over and was not heard from again.[10]

Although the structured activities of the group (i.e. the relaxation and meditation) largely downplayed the kind of social interactions that might normally be associated with support groups, it is not to be supposed that these were completely absent. In fact, it is simply that they occurred in a much more informal and *ad hoc* way than was observed in other groups – largely as unplanned satellite encounters. The physical setting of the group – at the heart of the cancer hospital – and the day-to-day presence of the organiser in her ongoing role as a CAM provider meant that there were many opportunities for informal interactions which did not happen directly as a result of 'formal' group meetings. A good example of this is the way in which, following sessions, most participants who were able to would meet up in the hospital café. In a sense, these informal meetings were a direct extension of group activities and provided an arena where any extra post-session 'debriefing' could be engaged in. From our observations it was evident that this was exactly what some participants used them for. Significantly, even though she encouraged new members to join in with them, the therapist deliberately avoided attending these gatherings herself, reporting that she could see benefits in allowing members space to express themselves without having to worry about what she might think.

At a wider level, too, the physical geography of the area around where the therapist worked encouraged extra-group encounters. Due to her treatment room being only big enough to accommodate three or four people (the therapist, a patient on the couch and a seat for a carer), a space at the side of the communal area had been appropriated as a place where patients and other stakeholders could wait (see Figure 4.1). Over a number of years, this space had developed into a small library of CAM-related books, and had a collection of therapeutically themed videos (such as guided meditations) which patients could watch on a small video player. Everything in the library area had been donated by patients or the therapist, and it contained an eclectic mix of material ranging from books on cancer and cancer care, through to pamphlets on esoteric and borderline quack therapies.[11] 'Official' information leaflets dealing with cancer and CAM treatments were also displayed. What is interesting about the library is the fact that it acted as an informal 'drop-in' centre. Even when the therapist was not on hand, or was giving a treatment in her room, patients could be found browsing or chatting in the library area. It essentially acted as a kind of ongoing group meeting in which information was exchanged, and contacts maintained. The therapist also made active use of the library area as a means of informally socialising with patients – regularly coming out of her room to see who was there, introducing herself and offering information about the group. She reported that patients and others who were interested in learning more about healing, but who were perhaps not quite ready to commit to a session, sometimes found their way into the library. This unthreatening environment acted as an ideal place to engage them and 'demystify' the CAM services on offer. Similarly, the therapist had received many positive testimonials from patients over the years, and she had bound these in two large scrapbooks which were on prominent display.

This location of interactional activities away from the focus of the group meeting itself has important implications for the propagation of CAM-related information. In other group settings – where formal CAM activities were usually balanced by feedback and discussion time with the CAM provider and/or group organisers – this process can be seen as being overly integrated as a discrete therapeutic activity. However, it is in effect limited by distinct temporal, locational and organisational boundaries; it only really takes place in the context of the 'formal' group setting. Extra-therapeutic and experiential interactions in the present example group are different. Despite their ostensive absence from the meditation and relaxation sessions themselves, they are in effect far more dynamic and allow for a greater range of interactions to take place. The multiple physical locations and contexts which are available to participants around this group (but which still retain 'group' connections) mean that restrictions encountered in one setting can usually be overcome in another. If, for example, a patient attending a group session wished to discuss something, but did not necessarily want to do it in front of the group itself, they could utilise one of the other settings where co-members or the therapist might be found (the library, or at the informal post-group café meetings, for example).

The propagation of CAM-related information during the group sessions themselves was a more contentious issue. The therapist, and the majority of people who came to meetings, were by definition at least interested in approaches to healing which were outside of those used by biomedicine. The fact that the group was being operated from within a biomedically dominated healthcare system, and by a therapist who was in the pay of this system (albeit tenuously), therefore created noticeable difficulties when it came to the kinds of information that could be discussed at meetings and disseminated by the therapist. While there were no formal restrictions placed on the group by the hospital, it was evident on several occasions that the therapist carefully avoided being drawn into discussions that might have been contentious, or which might have undermined her position. A topic which cropped up relatively frequently in the pre- and post-session interaction was the efficacy or otherwise of biomedical treatments over CAM, and the use of various herbal preparations. Whenever the therapist was put in a position where she had to comment on these, she would emphasise that what she was offering was *complementary* to biomedical cancer treatments, and could not replace them.[12]

In this chapter we have used the backdrop of a detailed group activity case study to introduce issues and processes which are relevant to a wide range of different group types and organisational approaches. We have drawn together both structural and interactional elements, and examined the complex interrelations between the two. It is clear that the cancer support group environment occupies an idiosyncratic position in relation to both biomedical healthcare services and CAM, and that this has numerous important impacts on the everyday practicalities of service provision. Factors that in other medical support settings might not be significant (such as the particular belief systems that inform the approaches of key organisers and therapists) can take on a new resonance. Issues relating to how stakeholders interpret and utilise information on CAM, for example, generate a whole raft of interactional issues which simply do not exist in biomedical arenas; biomedical cancer care does not require or incorporate 'belief' in the same way that much of CAM does (or may appear to), and once there is even a tenuous spiritual dimension to proceedings, achieving an environment that does not exclude or alienate certain individuals is very difficult.

At a broader level, we have tried to show how tensions can arise between location and the enactment of CAM processes – particularly when the setting for group activities is closely tied to a hospital or other biomedical environments. In these settings organisers are not only required to deal with the ubiquitous tensions of the CAM/biomedical dynamic; they are also required to utilise spaces in which they are essentially outsiders or, at best, hold marginal status – something which can actually be very constructive in terms of improving integration awareness, but which (as in the case of our main example) may equally have the effect of deepening mistrust and misalignment.

Another source of tension connected with the practicalities of organising a support group is related to the 'open access' policy operated by the majority of such organisations. This operates in two ways. On one level most groups encourage non-patients (i.e. carers) to participate in activities alongside patient members. This kind of open access appears to have little impact on the practical provision of CAM within or by a group, and is usually considered beneficial, both for patients and carers. Where open access can be more troublesome is where it relates to the accommodation of new and 'CAM inexperienced' members alongside individuals with much greater CAM-related knowledge. In this case, it appears that the structural adaptations required in order to maintain inclusion can have a slight, but noticeable effect on the depth (if not the quality) of CAM provision; rather than following a trajectory in which members presumably get better and better at a given activity (say, meditation), the regular appearance of neophyte members effectively means that a great deal of basic groundwork is constantly being re-presented at the expense of more advanced activity. This is, of course, limited to those forms of CAM which – as in our main example – are wholly enacted at a group level. It cannot be said to be a significant problem at the individual level (i.e. one-to-one sessions).

Chapter 5

Confined innovation

Organisational challenge
and its limitations

In Chapters 3 and 4, we provided an outline of the structural and interactional elements which underpin CAM/cancer support group environments. In this chapter we move the analysis one stage further – to an examination of the extent to which CAM/cancer support groups are (and are able to be) operationalised in such a way as to provide something innovative, and ultimately, to be a challenge to the therapeutic and organisational 'mainstream'. In so doing we take full account of the 'confined' location (therapeutic and geographical) in which such groups exist. By this we refer to the difficult, and frequently marginal, spaces that they occupy, spaces which we have described in-depth in earlier chapters. While the rhetoric of innovation (i.e. of offering something that questions the status quo) may form a part of the backdrop to group-based CAM provision, questions remain about the extent to which this can be and is translated into practice at a grassroots level. We will approach this task by looking at three aspects of support group structures and processes: 1) the nature of formal and informal gatekeeping in groups – how this affects group composition and is influenced by structural constraints; 2) the extent to which 'challenge' is discernible in the way groups are constituted and organised; 3) the extent to which broader inequalities are challenged by groups.

In the first part of this chapter, then, we will focus on the role that key individuals play in determining the direction and ethos of support group environments. This is of some significance because of the frequently marginal and ambiguous status of groups at the point of intersections between professional and lay, and between CAM and biomedicine. As noted above, central to our analysis is the concept of 'gatekeeping'. In the context of this study, gatekeeping (and the individuals who overtly or covertly perform this role) is particularly salient. Like any other area of healthcare, there are specific routes along which individuals are guided (subtly and not so subtly) as they navigate disease and treatment processes. At a basic level, gatekeeping may be reflected in interactions with the receptionist at a patient's local GP surgery, or the secretary of their oncologist; actors who attempt to filter out potentially difficult encounters on the behalf of their employer (i.e. doctors). In the context of CAM/cancer support groups, however, gatekeeping becomes a more complex and opaque issue. Aside from the purely functional administrative gatekeeping that might occur in any group or organisation, there can also be deeper structural dimensions to such processes. For in this situation there is a crucial role to be played in determining which therapies and therapeutic perspectives patients are introduced to – a process that is pivotal in setting the terms of reference for patient engagement with what constitutes CAM in any given situation.

To begin with, therefore, our attention is centred on those aspects of support group development and organisation that particularly relate to the individualistic and structural influence of different types of gatekeeping. We will examine how informal and formal gatekeeping shapes both the context and content of support group activities, and explore how the overt or unconscious imposition of certain CAM perspectives by advocates and organisers tends to underlie the entire CAM/cancer support group arena. We will argue that, contrary to what might be expected, the drive towards acceptance and incorporation embraced by many grassroots and independent groups has resulted in stronger and more multilevel gatekeeping in these types of organisation – processes which contribute to the delimiting of radical innovation in the nature of therapeutic practice.

Gatekeeping and the provision of CAMs in support groups

Problems

The day-to-day management of a cancer support group – even a small informal organisation – can be a significant challenge. As with any group, there will be the complex organisational and interpersonal dynamics (and disputes), as well as a range of administrative duties, to cope with. Unlike many other organisations, however, stakeholders in the CAM/cancer field operate in a disease context charged with a high degree of emotional turmoil. Most of the patients involved in such groups will be seriously ill, and a significant proportion will die while still members of the group. This poses real challenges to participants and organisers in terms of balancing mourning processes versus ensuring the group is positive and supportive for the participants who are still alive. For CAM-based cancer support groups there are even more inherent difficulties. On the one hand, such groups are essentially dealing with the provision of a therapeutic service which (depending on the actual CAMs being offered) is likely to be, at the very least, contentious – particularly as viewed by the biomedical community. This potentially alienates an organisation from a large proportion of the stakeholders (i.e. biomedical health professionals) who might be in a position to help them recruit patients and operate the group effectively. On the other hand, a key issue in these groups is where to draw the line in terms of which CAMs to provide or sanction, and just how 'alternative' they can afford to be. As we have explored already, groups that espouse the rejection of biomedical cancer treatment tend to become self-limiting in terms of the level of membership they can hope to maintain. In actuality, they tend to end up cutting themselves off from the well established health networks, and in doing so, alienate those who are the gatekeepers to patient access and 'professional legitimacy'.

Advocacy and constraint

Another aspect of this multifaceted environment, which is, by definition, central to the delivery of therapies, is, of course, the therapists and individual advocates who actually try to provide them in these group environments. These individuals understandably seek to make the services they offer available to as many people as possible (this is generally a product of both a belief on the part of the therapist that CAMs are effective, combined with a desire to promote their therapeutic practice). For these advocates, the issue of acceptability to the 'mainstream' takes on a very different meaning. While they may well realise the necessity of 'falling in line' with biomedical cancer networks to some degree (and the subordination of their therapeutic practices that often results within 'partnerships' with biomedical professionals), they are also likely to perceive themselves as more than just another facet of contemporary cancer care (such as some may perceive a nurse, for instance). As advocates and providers of an 'alternative' to biomedical cancer treatment they will have generally invested a great deal of energy in establishing themselves as 'outsiders'. They will spend a high proportion of their professional life defining their approach as something that is essentially different from the methods of biomedicine, and which only they, as CAM therapists, have the time and inclination to capitalise on.

> I suppose most people who come have an inclination that it's going to be different even if they haven't, you know, had [CAM] before, so most people are used to a bit more of a conventional style. I think they recognise it is a different thing – they haven't got to get through it all in ten minutes or whatever ... you get a better angle on what it is that's troubling someone. So obviously you need to know what it is that brings them to you, but just what it is may not be quite so defined as what you might first think. There might be a whole set of things, maybe a whole range of difficulties, or challenges or whatever. So it may be quite a complex pattern and people will elaborate, so it's not always a tight process ... If somebody came with a migraine, say, I mean, I would

probably spend about 20 minutes talking about the migraine and the other one hour ten minutes talking about everything else – and even in a follow-up [consultation] it would be the same ...

(CAM therapist, homeopath, Group 4)

As biomedical knowledge and expertise comes under increasing public scrutiny (and public interest in CAM increases), an 'alternative' yet 'professional' approach can serve as a useful marketing tool (a strategy of delineation and self-promotion within the cancer services). In the context of cancer support groups, however, it may not be so helpful. CAM providers and therapists are clearly key components of any CAM-focused organisation, but these groups will almost certainly want to attract patients who are already immersed in biomedical disease and treatment processes. These individuals will often already be enmeshed in biomedical health networks and generally will be strongly backing whatever biomedicine can offer (and often, so too will their carers and families). Thus, unlike many other types of CAM-based self-help groups (i.e. groups simply focused on self-development and general wellbeing), groups providing CAM for cancer patients are working in an area that places them in direct contact (and sometimes even conflict) with the positivist and medico-reductionist foundations of biomedical cancer care. To remain viable entities (i.e. at least loosely connected with other biomedical cancer services) they tend to place restrictions on the level of 'alternative' rhetoric they espouse – at least in public.

At college we were told that we would very rarely, if ever, see anyone who had just opted for the alternative and they would normally say, 'I've had chemo, I've had radiotherapy, I've had everything they've offered me. Can you do something as well?' And it's like everything that's offered to them they will take and out of fear, and yet you see, I have people coming to me saying, 'I've been told that the cancer has gone away now, but they are just going to offer me some more chemo – just in case – and I've said, yes please, yes please.' You know and it's just fear, isn't it ...

(CAM therapist, homeopath, Group 4)

Everything's a lot tighter now. It's not as airy-fairy as it was ten years ago. If you work in those kinds of places [hospitals] you've really got to be careful. You can't go on about angels and spirits – even if it's what you believe. You have to be careful who might get to hear about it and get the wrong idea ... I know doctors who understand about these things, but they'd never admit to it ... it's a shame really.

(CAM therapist, healer, Group 5)

The tension between gatekeeping and advocacy

Gatekeeping in relation to cancer support groups and CAM operates in a number of ways. There is, of course, the channelling of patients away from CAM by biomedical health professionals (either subtly or explicitly) who express little interest in what different therapeutic modalities might have to offer. However, explicit gatekeeping by biomedical staff, although still occurring, has become less politically savvy in a sociopolitical context whereby policies espousing integration are increasingly visible. Recognition of public support for CAM and the apparent value of certain CAM practices (e.g. acupuncture and relaxation therapies) have led to more reluctance on the part of biomedical clinicians to dismiss CAM approaches openly. However, it seems clear that more sophisticated forms of gatekeeping still operate in some biomedical contexts which allow clinicians to channel their patients away from many CAM services (for further discussion see Broom and Tovey, forthcoming).

Support for integration within the biomedical community can itself be seen in these terms: as an evolving process of professional regrouping. The current move towards the adoption of integrative practice opens up new points of contestation about who has the power to shape the relationship between CAM and biomedicine. In the face of approaches that can go well beyond the purely medical to incorporate elements of spirituality, lifestyle choice and sociopolitical awareness, the simplistic and ineffective response of outright rejection initially adopted has now been superseded by varying degrees of appropriation and incorporation. Such 'integration' on the terms of those with existing power is of course very different from any notion of a coming together of differing paradigms within a neutral environment.

However, while it is important to recognise the political context for action and the potential gain for particular professional groups of adopting specific strategies, this should not lead to a simplistic view that there are no serious issues to be addressed about the role of CAMs in the context of cancer care. There are, for instance, concerns about the regulation of CAMs, and the efficacy and economic viability of the provision of such treatments in UK cancer services which cannot be reduced to concerns about the diminution of professional authority alone. These are concerns generated through a means of assessing practices which (in theory) permeates biomedical provision. While, of course, the evidence base for many established procedures is scant, the consensus on the way to evaluate practices (through the generation of 'evidence') is nonetheless pervasive.

The situation is, then, a little more complex than is sometimes presented – being rather more nuanced than previously represented by many biomedical clinicians on the one hand, and CAM advocates on the other. Indeed, even with the rather volatile positioning of CAM in relation to biomedicine, in the context of a high profile disease like cancer, so-called 'responsible' gatekeeping has evolved within the CAM movement itself, and is therefore evident within patient support groups that have an active CAM component. In such contexts there is growing awareness that CAM practitioners (and their advocates) need to project the impression that they are capable of (and are currently achieving) effective forms of self-regulation. We suggest that because of this, gatekeeping in such organisations has become quite rigorous. Groups that need to develop or maintain close links with biomedical cancer networks appear to work very hard at demonstrating that they are 'worthy' of mainstream credentials. That is, they have stringent procedures in place which are often apparently quite restrictive. They enthusiastically vet, test, monitor and evaluate anyone who might want to join the support group, and like to demonstrate to 'outsiders' (particularly biomedical clinicians who act as gatekeepers) that they can spot and exclude a 'flaky therapist'.

> When people [therapists] apply to come here, they ring up and say they want to volunteer for maybe, reflexology or aromatherapy, or whatever, so we need first of all to look at their qualifications and the training that they have had and make sure that that is of a standard that is acceptable to organisations like the Aromatherapy Organisation Council or I am a member of the International Federation of Professional Aromatherapists. It is quite thorough, and then you have to go on to post-grad training and most of them here have done extra courses in cancer care and things like that as well. So what happens is we look at the training they have had, then they come down and have an interview with the Director and myself and we talk to them about the suitability of working with cancer patients, and their own experiences at looking after anybody with cancer, and then they are asked to perform demonstrations so we can judge their reaction and how they cope with that. Then if that's OK then we get to references, and if that's OK then they start with me and come in and observe two or three sessions. Then I observe them for the same amount of time and then they are let loose ... We are not aiming to treat anybody, our main aim is to support them while they are undergoing treatment or if they have had treatment, so we make very clear that they [prospective therapists] know never to try and change other people's ideas on their treatment at all.
>
> (Organiser, Group 5)

CAM, as we have pointed out previously in this book, is not a cohesive collection of therapies working together to forward the cause of 'holism' or 'naturalism'. It is an intensely compartmentalised and eclectic mix of (often competing) therapeutic modalities, each with their own ontological and epistemological perspectives on the nature of disease and illness. Similarly, different therapies engender significantly varied degrees of credibility within the CAM 'movement' itself. There are relatively professionalised therapies at one extreme (such as homeopathy and acupuncture) and practices which remain marginal (even within the CAM community) at the other. These might include practices such as crystal healing or other esoterically focused activities. Such therapies – which could be viewed as representing the two extremes on the continuum of CAM modalities – still vary substantially on matters of regulation, professionalisation and institutional support.

The project of integration – or pressures put on CAM by stakeholders within this project – therefore encourages a degree of self-regulation from CAM providers themselves (at least, from those who place any value on the process of integration). The organisers of CAM support groups are keenly aware that it is in their interests to limit explicit critiques of biomedicine and the espousal of the more alternative discourses of illness, the body or medicine. This is particularly the case if groups (or group organisers) aim to utilise reflected authority (gained from an association with biomedicine) as a means of legitimising the services they offer.

At one level, then, it may be through the indirect gatekeeping undertaken within groups (to appease biomedical authority) that some of the apparent restrictions on CAM actually develop. If a group, for example, can demonstrate that it chooses not to provide anything too 'radical' or contentious by way of CAM therapies, it will be less concerned about alienating biomedical health professionals who are the gatekeepers to patient access. This is why in the cancer groups we are exploring, CAM is only operationalised in limited terms. Within the context of cancer care, the integration that is occurring is very limited in terms of the practices offered and is largely ideologically tame (i.e. the more benign and soft CAMs are more likely to be offered to cancer patients). Thus, the dynamics we analyse here at the sites where selected CAMs are being integrated should only be viewed as a glimpse of what the wider integration of CAM could engender. In cancer care, CAM can effectively become defined by a few 'safe' therapeutic modalities.[13] This can be seen across incorporated and independent organisations. It is only in the more extreme 'grassroots' support groups that the 'harder' more 'invasive' CAMs are introduced to, and potentially used by, patients.

In the majority of independent support organisations where CAM services are available, the individuals who most readily take on gatekeeping roles are therefore likely to be therapists, or individuals who have a vested interest in the provision of certain types of CAM. When deciding who is 'in' and who is not, they need to consider what is good for the continued viability of the group, as well as any preferences they may have regarding the underlying credibility of what is proposed. In some cases where relations with biomedical networks are tenuous, or where professional standing is perceived to be threatened, they may also need to consider how the involvement of other (possibly less 'integrated') therapists might reflect on their position. In groups with a direct NHS affiliation, however, the situation is likely to be more straightforward. Although issues of safety (i.e. the safety of treatments) are important to groups of all types, in organisations that have strong links to the mainstream, the dynamic appears to be very much skewed towards *protection from*, rather than *provision of*, CAM. It is often evident that regardless of the apparent openness with which some incorporated groups embrace CAM, the underlying dynamic is one of fear – fear that what they offer will harm patients and undermine the 'real' treatments they are being given.

The opening part of this chapter has been concerned with the role that advocates and gatekeepers play in facilitating access to CAM in the cancer support group arena. We argue that the nature of the cancer field places individuals who perform key roles in a unique and challenging position. On the one hand they may wish to push forward with the 'project' of CAM integration, but on the other they face restrictions which are both self-imposed and generated as the result of ongoing tensions with the biomedical community. The practical reasons for certain CAM modalities being more common than others in cancer care have also been explored. In addition it can be noted that along with issues of self-imposed and external gatekeeping, some CAM therapies are unsuitable for use in a group environment (that is, they are fundamentally tied to the 'one-to-one' patient–practitioner encounter). This has meant that, for organisations that are set up to provide improved access to CAM, practical issues related to supply come into play, and comparatively individualistic approaches (in terms of the number of people who can access a treatment during a given session) often give way to more collective therapies. This dynamic is particularly evident in newly forming organisations where maximum access for minimum cost is paramount.

Organisational challenge and innovation

As we have illustrated thus far, the supposedly innovative and revolutionary aspects of the CAM movement are only expressed within support group environments in a limited way (at least, in terms of the kinds of therapies which they espouse). However, we were also interested in exploring whether there is evidence of paradigmatic and ideological innovation being expressed in the underlying structures of organisations – particularly in those groups which have an overt CAM ethos (i.e. Type 2 groups). The extension of holistic ideals into the mechanics of how groups are organised and run is fundamental to the image of many organisations. And so we may ask such questions as: do groups provide an arena for innovative provision that may not otherwise be available? Can the interactional processes which the groups facilitate be seen as innovative therapeutic resources in their own right? And so on. Elements such as the rejection of conventional hierarchical group structures and the adoption of egalitarian methods of participation are routinely cited in the rhetoric of organisations as being very important to group members, and often form part of the expressed aims of groups.

> ... I'll facilitate – but I'm always checking with people, you know, nothing's written in stone, we can do it or not do it and because all of that seems to work, I'm not going to try and change it. Last time I suggested we bring food and share it ... say something like in the winter a bowl of soup and a roll and in the summer time some kind of salad or mixed fruit or whatever, and I suggested that we get a roster of who prepares and who serves, it's a gesture of we all take turns in giving and receiving, isn't it ... We are very good at giving sometimes but we are not all good at sitting there and accepting what people offer. It all comes back to being holistic, doesn't it?
>
> (Facilitator/Organiser, Group 4)

In our study, two of the Type 2 groups (Groups 3 and 4) were probably most representative of this kind of holistically grounded approach. Although these particular organisations were somewhat different, in that one (Group 3) was very well established, and the other was in its initial stages of development, a key commonality was the emphasis given to making the practicalities of membership as egalitarian as possible.

> ... you never get the feeling that somebody's in charge and organising things. You don't get the feeling you're sitting in the wrong chair or anything because you can get that with some people. No, it's very free and easy and open and everyone's on an equal footing. No one's got a specific role – I mean I'm on the committee, but I just sort of put in ideas, and it's more or less the way it works for all of us. Sometimes Anne [CAM therapist] will ask a particular member to do something but it's very, very open – there's no rigid structure, it's very easy-going and that seems to work.
>
> (Male group member, age 68, lung cancer)

The fact that 'anti-hierarchical' rhetoric is so often found in arenas where CAM practices are advocated and utilised reflects the extent to which these modalities intersect with the wider life world perceptions of those involved. Although ostensibly a therapeutic activity, CAM in the context of cancer support groups is rarely found in isolation – its presence in any environment tends to reflect broader social and organisational conventions, and can often be taken as an indication that there will be other aspects of the wider 'CAM project' just below the surface. Even in relatively conservative Type 1 settings (such as the hospital-based Group 8, where CAM provision was relatively minimal and consisted of occasional out-sourced movement-based therapies), it was evident that the therapeutic contact engendered had a wider influence. Patients who participated in CAM activities at this group, for example, appeared to carry over some of the 'holistic' ethos they had been experiencing during their (t'ai-chi) sessions into the regular 'non-CAM' activities of the group.

The underlying egalitarian nature of most holistic and CAM-related movements has a strong influence on the aims and objectives of groups. A key factor here is the facilitation of activities and environments that will be actively empowering to patients. This may simply be manifest at the level of enabling patients to engage with therapies and processes (i.e. CAMs) that lie outside of the jurisdiction of biomedicine, and so encourage them to feel that they have control over aspects of their treatment: when they utilise CAM modalities it is largely they who decide if and when they will explore a given therapy, repeat its use, or experiment with combinations of treatments. Similarly, whether or not they choose to tell their GPs and oncologists about what they are doing is their decision, and this too can encourage a sense of empowerment. This is particularly the case if a patient feels that he or she has exhausted all that biomedicine can offer. One group member talks about discussing their CAM use with their doctor:

> I don't think it is anything to do with them. I think they are there to deal with the medical side of things; that's their job, so I had a surgeon who did the surgery, and I had an oncologist who saw to the radiotherapy and the chemotherapy and the Tamoxifen drug treatment. I asked right at the beginning should I be eating anything different and they all said, 'Oh no, no', so I know they are not interested in that. And why should they be because they are doctors; they do the drugs. I think you have got to take control and do it yourself; you can't say, 'Oh the doctor didn't do this and the doctor didn't do that' – why should they? Just say, 'Thank you, doctor', and go and eat some flax seed or something.
>
> (Female, age 51, Group 4, breast cancer)

Significantly, it is within the patient support groups that have the most turbulent and fractured relationships with biomedical cancer networks (i.e. independent and support grassroots groups) that patient empowerment can be most evident. In organisations that are routinely at odds with aspects of biomedical cancer care, or where there has been a significant degree of isolation from, and struggle against, biomedical networks, a noticeable 'us' and 'them' culture can develop. Far from being counter-productive, at a basic level this outlook can actually be of significant benefit to a group. It allows a process of 'rallying together' for a common cause, helping to strengthen the self-identity of the organisation and produce greater cohesion amongst its members.

For a large number of cancer patients, association with a support group may well be the first contact they have with any form of CAM or holistically derived activity. So, in this context it could be said that these groups as a whole are indeed providing an important resource – a significant means by which the all-important first connections with CAM are established. Whether or not this pathway to CAM is particularly significant in terms of wider provision, however, is questionable. Although the throughput of cancer patients attending support groups and engaging with CAM does technically form a large and diverse sample, they are still only a small and select proportion of the population at large, and the limited range of therapies they access (at least on an 'official' level), does not accurately reflect dynamics between the wider CAM community and biomedicine. Cancer patients are similarly a relatively insular grouping. Given the narrow focus of motivation which grounds their involvement – their limited energies are usually channelled solely into their personal engagement with CAM – the activities of discrete groups will not necessarily have any significant impact outside of their particular membership base. Even evangelical enthusiasm for CAM in this context is only ever likely to reach other stakeholders connected with cancer in some way.

A final (and perhaps surprising) way in which patient support groups are indirectly facilitating CAM integration and therefore arguably a form of innovative practice is through the tangential access that they offer to biomedical health professionals. A significant number of GPs and other health professionals do have an interest in what CAM has to offer, but are seemingly reluctant to engage with it directly (by training as therapists, or providing therapies themselves, for instance). There are still relatively frequent reports of doctors being disciplined for providing overtly 'alternative' treatments (see, for example, Sheldon 2006) and this undoubtedly has the effect of discouraging involvement. By becoming connected with the activities of a patient support group, however, individuals are able to engage with CAM indirectly – particularly if the group has the legitimacy of being affiliated to the NHS. This kind of indirect contact allows biomedical practitioners to maintain a degree of professional distance from CAM whilst also engaging with their patients' interest and usage of CAMs. Nurses and allied health professionals also appear to utilise support groups in this way. Nurses, for example, are a professional group that is well represented in our data. Many group originators, organisers and CAM therapists have a nursing background, although the dynamic here is often slightly different to that of doctors. Recent research examining nurses who utilise CAM (Tovey and Adams 1999), for instance, has highlighted how for some nurses, or more specifically those most vocal in the advocacy of the incorporation of CAM into nursing, the appropriation of a 'CAM identity' becomes a means of 'escape' from the restrictions of professional subordination. It is very rare, however, to come across a doctor who gives up their biomedical creden-tials to embrace CAM.

However, although the rhetoric of innovation is present and examples of this are evident, as will now be shown, there was a consistent sense of this innovation being delimited and constrained – a consequence of the confined environment.

The membership structure of groups produces an interesting impact on the potential for innovation. Continuity of membership is an ongoing prob-lem for cancer support organisations and can be seen as having both positive and negative influences on the workings of a group. On the positive side, a well established membership base has an obvious stabilising effect; certain members will become 'fixtures' and embodiments of group identity. The group will have a stable base and project an element of permanence. On the negative side, however, such a deep-rooted membership can have a stifling effect on the ability of the group to adapt to new demands and processes. New members can feel as if they have to follow the established ways of the group and fit in with the implicit hierarchy. This can create entrenched patterns in interpersonal dynamics and facilitate a movement away from the potentially egalitarian ethos that may have driven the origi-nal emergence and development of the group. The management of entrenched members can be a troublesome issue for group facilitators – so much so that the sensitive handling of interpersonal relations is a serious challenge in groups where numbers may be small. The arguments, squab-bles and misalignments which are part of any group project are all the more damaging when turnover of members is restricted.

It also seemed that as some groups developed, the evolution of the approach of the organiser or facilitator had the effect of delimiting group dynamics and negatively impacting on the attempts of groups to maintain an open and holistic approach to group support (and their innovative char-acteristics). For example, a patient at one of our study sites reported difficulties that had arisen due to misalignments with a facilitator who had originated and run the group for a number of years, and who was closely identified with it.

> ... she becomes very possessive of her patients, and that's what hap-pened to me. It wasn't the [CAM therapy] I was against, it was the situation – she became very possessive and I had to just claw myself away because it wasn't helping me. There were a lot of issues around that, and if you didn't turn up it was, 'Where are you – where have you been?' I couldn't handle that.
>
> (Female group member, age 34, Group 1, breast cancer)

CAM-based support groups, then, are certainly not immune from the rou-tine problems of hierarchy and positioning which emerge in any multiparty environment. Even if they overtly espouse a non-hierarchical and egalitarian approach to organisation (as many groups do) the practicalities of achieving this and maintaining it over time are challenging. This seems particularly true for cases where some group members do not necessarily 'buy into' the overt rejection of conventional (and often hierarchical) group management structures in the same way as their more 'liberal' associates.

In part, such complex group dynamics emerge from the nature of the membership pool from which cancer support groups can expect to recruit, an eclectic and perhaps disparate range of individuals who often only have a cancer diagnosis in common. The kinds of people who may choose to attend a CAM-based group, or try out a CAM therapy, are not necessarily going to be 'political' in their perception of, or decision to utilise, CAM. Innovation in ethos and paradigmatic pluralism is thus difficult to achieve in contexts where world views differ considerably between group members. Our data suggests that even in groups where the rejection of hierarchical structures is part of the underlying rhetoric, these ubiquitous elements of social organisation tend to develop anyway, making the achievement of a truly 'holistic' environment extremely difficult.

It also emerged from our research that groups which actively avoid having any form of 'leadership' may very quickly lose direction, and, after an initial spurt of enthusiasm, tend to dissolve as members become disillusioned with the lack of organisational structure. The problem is not so much that people dislike the idea of egalitarian arrangements, it is more that without some form of leadership the peculiarities of sustaining a group in the CAM/cancer arena quickly throw up practical problems which, by their nature, demand that someone actually take charge and organise things.

> We all sat down and talked about what we wanted [from the new group] and we had a meditation and we had some strawberries and some juice and it was all very nice. I don't know whether they are wanting it to be a place that people can go and sit and talk – they have plenty of therapists but it needs organising. It does need somebody to get up there and organise it or it is just going to die down and it would be a shame because they are very nice people ... I think unless somebody else comes in who has a bit of get up and go it's just going to fall apart.
>
> (Female group member, age 60, Group 4, stomach cancer)

Thus, innovative group structures may be ideologically desirable but are frequently not practically achievable. This, it would seem, is embedded in the nature of the cancer support environment (an eclectic range of perspectives), but also the wider tendencies of hierarchical structures to develop in group contexts.

In this section we have considered the problems for CAM provision that arise within support groups that attempt to be explicitly egalitarian and holistic. It is evident that even more isolated, less 'mainstream' grassroots organisations are largely tied to established and conventional organisational structures; that is, if they desire longevity. It also seems the case that most patients attending a cancer support group where CAM is provided are not necessarily concerned with the wider political implications (in terms of the biomedical–complementary dynamic) of their CAM activities. A consequence of this is that too much pressure from organisers to develop 'radical' group structures (particularly ones that downplay the importance of some form of leadership) can, at times, severely limit membership and perhaps even result in the group being disbanded.

A challenge to health inequalities?

The third and final area of 'confined innovation' to be examined here is that relating to a potential challenge to health inequalities. Much of the rhetoric surrounding CAM positions it as a means of redressing the power imbalances which reportedly pervade biomedical activities. This function basically manifests itself on two levels. First, there are broad issues of patient choice over treatment options. CAM as a whole is usually represented as a movement which engenders self-determination for patients. Whereas biomedicine (and particularly the highly technologically based treatment processes which relate to diseases such as cancer) is largely about the use of expertise and established epidemiological knowledge to treat the patient, CAM treatments and therapies, on the other hand, have historically taken the approach of facilitating patient autonomy and empowerment in the process of healing.

> A lot of my friends who are on the periphery of the medical profession and have since left, they have been enthusiastic and they have found a fair amount of rejection or distancing – or that's what they have suggested anyway. And the other thing in this system is that if you get a doctor that you get on with, that's great, but it isn't systemic somehow. You're lucky if you get one that you connect with, especially if you've got kind of an alternative angle on things.
>
> (Female, age 63, Group 5, brain tumour)

Although many CAM modalities are still heavily reliant on expert providers (i.e. trained therapists), most offer a great deal more opportunity for self-medication by users. Once again, this emerges as particularly evident in the context of cancer or other illnesses which require the carefully controlled use of powerful prescription drugs. Even modalities such as homeopathy that are relatively 'therapist dependent' are open to experimentation, the remedies and preparations central to their operation being easily obtained by users without prescription. Information aimed at perpetuating this self-help culture is similarly widely available in many forms, from books and videos to DVDs and websites.

The second level at which CAM could be said to be challenging health inequalities relates more to individual interactions. More specifically, it can be said that the interactions that occur between CAM therapists and their patients are generally perceived to be more individualistically focused than those within biomedical consultations. A major appeal of CAM, for example, is the supposedly superior quality of the interpersonal interactions which occur between therapist and patient (Chatwin and Collins 2002). Aside from any actual curative or therapeutic effects that modalities themselves may or may not have, the CAM consultation is often represented as being a completely different experience from that enacted between a doctor and patient – even if the elements that go to create this experience may be difficult to describe.

> I don't know how you'd measure things like that ... I think you could very well end up with a clinical test that was negative and yet people still benefitted hugely [from CAM treatments] – I'm sure that happens. I think that simply the difficulty of setting up a test for something that's – it's not like testing a drug, is it? That you can measure chemically and come up with nice little figures. I don't know how you'd do it because surely there's the qualitative factor ... It may simply be the fact that doing something different rather than it being a particular activity – it's hard to pin it down.
>
> (Female group organiser and patient, age 56, Group 3, stomach cancer)

The indefinable 'human' qualities of CAM interactions continue to act as a draw for patients despite the fact that the process of professionalisation and integration has inevitably meant that much of the structural activity associated with the conventional 'medical encounter' have to some degree been appropriated. This is not to suggest that biomedicine is somehow compromised by its approach to patients, although many in the CAM world would undoubtedly argue that this is the case. Rather, it is to acknowledge that the cutting-edge treatments such as those used in cancer care are by their very nature going to preclude the kind of human contact in which many CAM therapies are grounded.

Beyond these elements that form the core of the rhetoric of CAM advocacy is a further area that receives limited attention but is one which actually represents an important dynamic in the way CAM is accessed and utilised across richer countries – that of gender.

Most usage information on CAM in the West suggests that although it may now be developing a broad appeal across all sectors of society, the largest and most active group of users are still white, middle-class and female. This characteristic has been borne out by the demographic make-up of the support organisations we worked with: all but one of our case study groups were started, run and organised by women, and had women providing the overwhelming majority of therapeutic services (see Chapter 2 for a more detailed description of the make-up of specific groups). It was evident in the accounts of the group members and organisers that use of CAM (and its delivery) tended to be a predominantly feminine pursuit.

> I think there are more men coming into it now as they train, but it is seen as more of a women's thing. And the men involved tend to be people who do physical things like osteopaths or yoga teachers – something like that. You get the occasional male healer and that's about it ...
>
> (Organiser, Group 8)

The only exception in our study was the internet-based support network aimed at prostate cancer sufferers (Group 7). This group dealt with a gender-specific cancer and naturally catered mainly for men. It was organised by, and attracted, participants who were almost exclusively male, although because the group was essentially an open-access internet forum it was difficult to ascertain how many female carers and relatives of prostate cancer sufferers took part as 'lurkers' (i.e. viewing the material posted on the site, but not posting messages). Occasional posts from women (usually carers of male sufferers) would appear, indicating that there was at least some active involvement, but these can not be taken as a true measure of the cross-gender appeal of the site. In this sense then, the environments we studied should not really be regarded as providing much in the way of structural evolution in respect of gender. CAM per se may be providing an active (though effectively indirect) means by which men's dominance of medicine is challenged, but this can perhaps be seen as another facet of polarisation rather than a significantly focused move towards a more egalitarian landscape. It appears that addressing the issue of gender inequality in the CAM/cancer support group context is not routinely a significant priority for stakeholders. Although the 'political' awareness of active individuals may have been sensitised by engaging with the wider sociomedical inequalities which surround CAM integration, groups are rarely initiated solely because of an awareness of the gender dynamic, or a wish to change it.

In terms of the more 'conventionally' organised groups in our study (i.e. those that actually held physical meetings) there was a similarly strong bias toward women's membership. Although none of our groups had an overt focus on cancers predominantly affecting women (such as breast cancer), women still dominated membership in all the sites we observed – two of the smaller groups having no male representation at all. Interestingly, however, no overt measures were observed in any of our groups to create a more representative user base (in terms of gender). The problem of gender bias among stakeholders, if it was addressed at all, tended to be regarded very much as a secondary and relatively unimportant issue. One group organiser talks about gender in relation to a group session:

> No, there were no male patients this week, but there was one man there and he was a homeopath, and he was very sensitive at the end. He addressed the group as a whole and said, 'I'm not feeling uncomfortable, but I want to put it to you that if anyone is uncomfortable and would like me to leave ...' and I thought that was really sensitive of him. And we all said no, and someone said we hadn't thought of it as 'male and female', we are just all here together ... When this guy brought this up we did then talk about what we wanted and the women there said, 'I think it would do men a lot of good to come, and to listen and to have a place to say, "This is scary", or whatever they feel. I think if we could get them through the door I think that would be OK ... It's just that there's still this stiff upper lip thing'.
>
> (Organiser, Group 4)

Of the relatively few men who are encountered in support group environments, a high proportion are likely to be carers rather than patients. These individuals are often brought along initially by their wives or partners (sometimes under some duress). Significantly, too, although they may initially be resistant to the kinds of 'emotionally enriching' approaches engendered by CAM, once they make the decision to become involved, it can be the men in the group who seem to get most from the experience. This can be particularly true of men who embrace meditative and relaxation practices. Several men who were group members in the study, for example, reported significant changes in their everyday lives after engaging with CAMs, such as meditation or healing. These types of therapy helping them to come to terms with tensions that had hitherto been repressed.

> ... my wife had just had her first chemo and we were on the floor. [The healing and meditation sessions] opened doors for us to relax, and to handle what was going on. Throughout the fourteen months of my wife's cancer, until she died in March this year, we came on a regular basis for holistic treatment, and we both found it very peaceful, very calming, very useful. It helped us through what was a very stressful, life-changing period. I still come [to the group] as much as I can, 'cos I get a lot of benefit ... When I first came [to a group session], I was a sceptic – I thought this is a load of twaddle. But I drifted off somewhere, and wherever I drifted off to, I had the sensation of my late father and my late brother holding my hand. They didn't say anything, but I knew it was them, and it shook me a bit. Then later, I must've gone really deep because they told me that I was howling like a dog with all the stress and tension that was built up in me, and the

meditation relieved that ... the reason I come [to the group] now is because of the solace it gives me, and my experiences in meditation have helped me get back on my feet. Though you never get over loved ones when they leave, it gives you strength to go on.

(Male group member, carer, age 46, Group 1)

What emerged was a common process by which men initially felt CAM approaches were rather more feminine pursuits, but after actually getting involved within the group context, they realised their potential for both men and women. This was particularly true of the 'soft' or 'airy-fairy' healing therapies which tended to be viewed as 'unnecessary'. However, it would also seem that men do struggle, at least initially, in support groups which are dominated by women, and choose not to participate rather than be a 'minority' within a group environment. Thus, we could not characterise support group processes as breaking down traditional gendered relations, or indeed, traditional patterns in access to CAM. However, they do potentially provide some access for men to get involved in CAM, and it would seem that in cases where men utilise this service, much is gained from their involvement.

Concluding comments

In this chapter we have addressed the issue of the extent to which the provision of CAM in cancer support groups can be regarded as innovative, or even as challenging to the status quo. In so doing, we considered the way in which gatekeeping practices and related processes shape a restricted operationalisation of therapeutic pluralism. We also considered the actual structure of groups and the impact of group activities on prevailing inequalities, with a particular focus on gender. On the basis of our research, we would argue that what is happening can at best be seen as a form of confined innovation. While specific examples of individual initiatives or types of therapy offered clearly need to be appreciated as reaching beyond what would otherwise be available, such action has to be seen within a structural environment which serves to delimit radicalism. Indeed, practices that extend what is offered, or how therapies are presented, beyond what can be accommodated within the dominant structure, are widely recognised as inducing threat to a group's existence. And the way in which provision is operationalised is influenced by a recognition of that.

It would appear, then, that much of the rhetoric that stresses the innovative and pioneering nature of the CAM 'project' is slightly misleading (in the context of cancer support groups at least). Support groups may indeed provide people with access to some forms of CAM, and are most certainly a means by which a large number of cancer patients first engage with 'alternative' perspectives on healthcare, but in the wider context of integration, the information and services that most support groups tend to focus on only represent a small part of the CAM field, and can not be said to be having a significant impact on entrenched biomedical positions. At a broader level, too, the actual mechanics of the majority of CAM/cancer support groups are not as innovative as perhaps they represent themselves; they rarely, for example, represent radical, innovative or experimental approaches to group structure, and those that do tend to be essentially self-limiting in terms of recruitment. Even radical 'grassroots' organisations which attempt to develop hierarchically free environments rarely manage to escape the practical restrictions faced by organisations operating in the 'real world'. As is the case with the consumption, integration or indeed, marginalisation of CAMs at a broader level, use of CAM in cancer support groups cannot be studied in a vacuum. Politics, power and personal and professional interests continue to impinge directly on developments.

Chapter 6

An exploratory comparative case study from Australia

Australia has followed a trajectory which is very similar to those of most other Western countries in terms of the growing popularity of CAM. As we outlined in Chapter 1, recent estimates indicate that Australians spend $1.8 billion a year on CAM (MacLennan *et al.* 2006), and that, as in other countries, the CAM services available to patients have grown significantly over recent years. The aim of this chapter is to present the results of the first exploratory case study of the provision of CAM in a cancer support group in Australia. We focus on one particular hospital-based support group positioned at the confluence between the biomedical system and the 'alternative' (i.e. being located in a hospital setting, but not forming part of the medical referral process). Our intention is to explore the extent to which the 'semi-official' position of this group influences the way in which it functions at both a formal and informal level, and to provide initial comparative data from a more affluent society that has a healthcare system which is different from that found in the UK. As outlined in Chapter 2, the case study approach was deemed to be the most effective in this context because it enabled us to incorporate data from a variety of sources. It also ensured that material gathered in Australia was methodologically compatible with that collected in the UK, thus maximising the potential for viable comparisons to be made. Thus, as was discussed in more detail in Chapter 2, we utilised three main sources of data:

- *Participant observation of group activities* (i.e. taking part in the structured meditation sessions that the group provided and the informal pre-/post-interactions within which these activities were embedded)
- *Qualitative interviews,* both informal and semi-structured, with group organisers, group members and other stakeholders
- *Document analysis,* including the analysis of publicity material by and about the group, reports, policy/intent statements, group handouts and other documentation such as internal evaluation questionnaires which the group utilised.

Key themes

Although this was essentially an exploratory study, we aimed to capture as complete a picture as possible of the group environment – its activities; its members; its position as part of the hospital where it was based; the dynamics of its location within the Australian sociomedical paradigm; and the extent to which it could be regarded as being a representative example of groups of this type. In particular, we wanted to be able to relate the data gathered directly to three of the main themes that had emerged in the UK data. First, there was the issue of *organisational structure*. Was the Australian group subject to different external and internal influences? Was it run or maintained in a significantly different way to other groups in our corpus? Did it stand out as being idiosyncratically Australian, or did the essentially Western health perspectives that underpinned its working arena mean that there were only superficial differences in approach and organisation? Similarly, we wanted to know about the level of *innovation* engendered by the group – both in terms of its role in CAM provision in the Australian context, and in terms of any broader sociopolitical influence it may reflect. As we have outlined already, our UK data has tended to indicate that far from being at the vanguard of revolutionary shifts in sociomedical development, CAM provision in most 'Type 1' support groups can be regarded as relatively non-threatening in relation to the biomedical 'mainstream'. In terms of its position on the Type 1/Type 2 continuum, our Australian group occupied a very similar position to the case study group presented in Chapter 4; it was something of a hybrid, operating from well within the established healthcare system, yet subtly distant from it. It was overt in its espousal of its complementary credentials, yet was run by healthcare professionals with key roles in the conventional organisation of the host hospital. What influence did this dynamic have on the ability of the group to provide innovation in terms of CAM and CAM provision? Indeed, would CAM innovation in the Australian context prove to be somewhat constrained as it turned out to be in the UK? Last, we wanted to concentrate on the issues of *gatekeeping* which had been highlighted in our earlier analysis. What kind of direct or indirect influence did the host hospital have over the way the group was run (in terms of CAM provision)? And further, what influence did the group organisers have? Was the CAM they championed a reflection of wider trends in the Australian CAM scene, and was this scene comparable to that found in the UK?

The meditation group

The Australian case study focused on a meditation and relaxation group based at the Coaltown Angel Hospital, one of three large public hospitals that serve a coastal region in New South Wales (NSW). The Angel is primarily known locally as a centre for oncology services and is the regional centre for services which include haematology, breast cancer screening, diagnosis and treatment, and melanoma diagnosis and treatment. It also offers a range of auxiliary and support services for cancer patients and their carers including occupational therapy, genetic counselling and various rehabilitation services. Interestingly, due to the fact that a significant proportion of the Angel's patients are drawn from outlying rural and remote areas, there are dedicated facilities to accommodate relatives and carers. This includes motel-type accommodation for which a small charge is made. The Angel also has a thriving volunteer organisation, the members of which can be identified around the hospital by their green badges. The volunteers play a key role in representing the hospital in the community, as well as helping to organise and run fund-raising events and awareness-raising initiatives.

Situated within the hospital grounds is the Graceland Hospice. This is affiliated to the palliative care service and provides pain and symptom management, short-term respite care and terminal care. Established in 1993, it is a purpose-built, 20-bed facility with large patient rooms that open out onto a landscaped communal courtyard. Care provided in the hospice offers people in the Coaltown area 'a choice which affirms life and all it has to offer, as well as understanding that dying is part of living.'[14] Admission requests to the hospice are made via a patient's local GP or specialist, and are considered by a committee consisting of a social worker and a medical officer.

The cancer support group at Angel hospital was chosen as a fieldwork site from a shortlist of five possible CAM/cancer groups in the NSW area. The main reasons for its inclusion were that it was relatively small; its provision of CAM was straightforward (i.e. it ostensibly focused on providing only one activity – meditation); its client base was largely drawn from the local area, which would simplify the logistics of interviewing group members; and it was structurally positioned within the mainstream Australian health system.

The degree to which this organisation can be considered to be representative of Australian groups in general is difficult to quantify. However, our preliminary investigations of the Australian CAM 'scene' revealed a situation very similar to that found in the UK, with a relatively high incidence of cancer support organisations per se, and a significant proportion of these offering at least some form of CAM – usually hands-on healing, massage or relaxation therapies. Another similarity was that the more esoteric or 'extreme' groups often appeared to be effectively isolated from mainstream health networks. So with this in mind, we decided to concentrate on a relatively 'mainstream' organisation – one in which there was likely to be a degree of active engagement between the group and established healthcare structures. Similarly, we hoped to find a group where the organisational structure involved a mix of biomedical health professionals and CAM providers, thus providing some insight into the dynamics of the interrelation between the two – something which might not be so readily observed in more 'grassroots' or independent settings where such encounters were less likely to occur.

Group structure and origins

The group was originally started in 1998 by two members of staff at the Angel – a social worker and an occupational therapist. These two individuals still organise and run the group, its activities forming an informal extension of their regular therapeutic roles. The organisers reported being motivated partly by a perceived need for this type of support service within the hospital, and partly because both had had positive experiences of selectively incorporating meditation into their therapeutic contact with cancer patients and their carers.

> ... occupational therapy has a really good history of using meditation and relaxation. It's something that we have exposure to – one of the professional skills that we use. We started doing it on the ward and we just found that there was quite a need for it. I thought, 'Well hey, why don't we start a group going?' So we started off the group, but at that stage it was on the ward and focused on relaxation.
>
> (Female group facilitator, occupational therapist)

The group is affiliated to the hospital to the extent that, after having been run regularly for several years, it was considered sufficiently established for a room to be made available for meetings. The fact that the organisers were well integrated members of the hospital staff undoubtedly helped in gaining access to this semi-permanent location, but even with the professional credibility that this brought, they reported occasional difficulties in this area. Unlike many UK sites, however, this apparently related to very practical issues of space and the difficulties of fitting in group activities alongside routine professional duties.

Publicity material advertising the weekly meditation sessions was relatively basic, and consisted of a photocopied leaflet which could be distributed to new patients, or picked up from reception where it could be found alongside the plethora of other health- and treatment-related information. Significantly, the primary information leaflet focused on meditation as the purpose of the group. This is interesting because in roughly equivalent UK groups, there appeared to be a reluctance to label CAM activities so overtly.

> Initially we were called a 'relaxation meditation group' because we thought just calling it a 'meditation group' would put off people and

putting the word 'relaxation' in might make it more accessible to people, but over the years that's something which changed. We realised that people are very happy to call it 'meditation'.

(Female group facilitator, social worker)

Publicity material for the meditation group carried the official hospital logo, and emphasised the connections with established healthcare networks. The role of the group as part of wider therapeutic services and support was emphasised, for example, as was the fact that the group facilitators had well established professional roles within the hospital. The style and design of publicity material was fairly basic and had a homemade feel. This was reportedly due to the fact that although the group was given a room to hold meetings, no direct funding was provided by the hospital as such; no money was available for materials such as refreshments for patients attending sessions, or other incidental items such as meditation mats for patients who may need to lie down, or tapes and CDs of meditation exercises that patients could take away. All of these items were provided to patients, but the money needed to supply them came from the occupational health facilitator's professional budget. This lack of funding was apparently a common problem, but again, it can be said to have very little to do with the specific CAM aims of the group. Antagonistic attitudes toward CAM provision, or hospital authorities withholding funds, were not a concern for this group, and neither is likely to be an issue in other similarly positioned organisations. Money for any type of extracurricular or 'non-essential' support activity in public health settings is *always* hard to come by. This is not a problem peculiar to the organisers of Australian support groups, and as was common in UK organisations, people would occasionally donate items, and anything of use was gratefully received.

Participation in the meditation sessions that formed the main work of the group was free and open to all oncology and haematology patients attending the Angel hospital and the Graceland Hospice. Carers and other stakeholders, such as health workers and medical staff, were also encouraged to attend, and during our period of fieldwork several carers came to the group, along with two former group members who had not attended for some time. These individuals had been given the 'all clear' or were in remission and no longer considered themselves to be 'cancer patients'. The benefit they derived from the incidental social support that the group offered, however, was sufficient for them to begin re-attending. This membership openness was another commonality with groups in the UK and highlights this apparently universal characteristic of cancer support groups.

The meditation group occupied a semi-official position within the hospital organisational structure and, as such, had no formal mechanism for patient referral. The main avenues by which patients found out about the group were the posters placed around the hospital, informal referral by hospital staff who knew about the group (and presumably valued it as a therapeutic resource) and information leaflets left in wards and waiting rooms. The group's semi-official status was further reinforced by the fact that it was not included in the list of support services routinely advertised in hospital literature. And similarly, although the hospital had an extensive website, there was no direct mention of the group or its activities, and no dedicated pages or links to CAM-related information and services.

Another key means by which people found out about the group was directly through the facilitators. Both of these individuals had regular professional contact with patients at various points during the time that they were being treated at the hospital, and when they judged that that involvement might be therapeutic (and, importantly, that a patient might be receptive), they would tell them about the group. Decisions regarding when, how, or if this should be done, however, were taken very seriously by the facilitators, and were reportedly informed by an in-depth knowledge of the underlying medical needs of the patient. This was particularly evident in relation to the possible contraindications that particular CAMs might have if they were used in conjunction with biomedical treatments such as radiation or chemotherapy. Even though the group offered a therapeutic service that was essentially neutral and non-reactive in biomedical terms, the facilitators were aware that patients who found an affinity with meditation might well develop an interest in other, more marginal, practices – ones that do not fit so well with the biomedical ethos or the approach of the hospital. It was clear from interviews with both group facilitators that they shared an interest and knowledge of CAM (and the attendant 'lifestyle' of health and spirituality which this knowledge often engenders) which went well beyond that which they shared with the group on a formal basis. As was the case with some of our UK Type 1 groups however, it was also evident that as individual interrelations between some group members and the facilitators developed, there was the likelihood that much more open sharing of experiences and CAM knowledge would take place. Essentially, it appeared that the facilitators felt that they needed to maintain a neutral and 'professional' persona until the position and receptivity of a given member in relation to CAM was assessed. In the following excerpt one of the group's facilitators talks about CAM therapies and recommending them to patients:

> I think that where I divide the line is that I don't see that it is possible for me to say to somebody who hasn't brought it up themselves, 'Why don't you try reiki or try this or that?' What I usually do is lead them into thinking about it by saying things like, 'Have you thought of anything else that might help you?' When they are deploring the state they are in I might say, 'What sort of other things might help?' and they will say,

'Well, so and so suggested this or that', you know, so I go into it that way; I would not bring it up and say, 'Why don't you ...' I mean, meditation I do bring up because I feel it has got a lot of credibility and it's not as touchy and it's not like suggesting they pay out heaps of money to go and have some treatment; they can come here [to the group] for free. So if people are indicating to me that they have stress and symptoms or whatever that might be helped by meditation I'm happy to bring that up by saying, 'Have you tried anything like that and would you be interested – would you like to have a sample of what it would be like?' But I would be cautious about bringing up herbal treatments or anything else myself – they would have to bring it up first.

(Female group facilitator, social worker)

The fact that the facilitators generally avoided drawing attention to their CAM activities, and basically treated the services that their group had to offer as pragmatic extensions of the therapeutic tools they routinely utilised (particularly in the case of the occupational therapist), suggests that they were very much aware of the limits of tolerance in terms of CAM and bio-medicine, and tailored their approach to incorporation with this very much in mind.

Group processes

As with the approach used in Chapter 4, the following discussion will be grounded in a description of an 'average' group meeting. This will be an effective way to illustrate some of the significant points which developed during the fieldwork and link these with our comparable UK observations. Each of the group sessions observed at the Angel conformed broadly to the format described here, and interview data with group members and facilitators confirmed that these were representative of routine meetings.

I Arrival of participants and informal talk period

Meditation group meetings were held every Thursday morning at 11.00 in a small room in the basement of the hospital. Sessions lasted around an hour, and although the nature of cancer treatment in a large hospital meant that synchronising sessions so that as many people as possible could attend was difficult, having a well established time and place for meetings was useful. Information posters advertising the group were left on display around the hospital, and on session days these doubled as way markers to the meditation room (with the addition of hand-drawn arrows).

For most of the time, the room where the group sessions were held was used as a general seminar and teaching space. On meeting days, however, the door was left open for half an hour or so before activities are scheduled to begin – the facilitators arranged the furniture in such a way that it was clear that a session was to be held. Facilitators were usually on hand during this pre-session period and it was normal for a trickle of regular members to arrive and utilise the time for informal socialising. If someone who was new to the group arrived, the facilitators were on hand to meet them and informally explain the workings of the session to them. This informal time was regarded as being very important by the facilitators – particularly as people encountering the group for the first time were likely to have differing expectations about the nature of what was going to occur.

As people arrived they usually took up a place on one of the ten or so chairs in the centre of the room (see Figure 6.1). These are arranged in a circle facing inwards. This arrangement is relatively ubiquitous in groups of this type (i.e. groups where meditation is an activity), and this is certainly the routine in the UK groups we studied (see Chapter 4). Interestingly, however, long-term members attending this group reported that when it first started, chairs had been arranged in rows facing the facilitators, and it was only at the suggestion of individuals who had attended other meditation-based groups that the circular positioning was adopted.

Once people were seated, the atmosphere was one of informal calm; facilitators chatted quietly to newcomers and informally explained what the group was for, what was going to happen, and what benefits it might have. The emphasis here was on the secular nature of meditation – how the exercises that the group performs may be regarded as purely physiological activities rather than anything religious or spiritual. If there were no new members present, this period usually developed into an informal group chat. Significantly, although cancer experiences and the swapping of stories related to ongoing treatment experiences were often observed by the researcher, CAM issues or anything tangentially related to these rarely appeared to be a topic of conversation at these times.

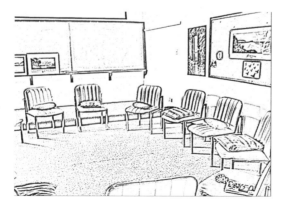

Figure 6.1 The meditation room

2 First guided meditation

Once a session was ready to begin, the facilitators indicated that the group should try to relax and become quiet – thus focusing attention on them as leaders of activity. When everyone was ready they then asked the group if there was any particular style of meditation they would like to work with that day. Unlike many other groups in our study, at the Angel there were a wide variety of meditation styles on offer ranging from relatively simple visualisations and breathing techniques, through to more esoteric routines which focused, for example, on particular colours or sounds as a means of stimulating healing. The type of meditation performed could therefore easily be tailored to the make-up and preferences of the group on any given day. However, the facilitators were consistent in their efforts not to display, or be seen to encourage, any particular religious content in the material that they utilised – a significant number of the relaxation and breathing techniques routinely performed, for example, were derived from medical, psychological and physiological sources rather than esoteric ones (e.g. neo-Buddhist practices). Both facilitators shared the job of 'guiding' the meditations and worked closely together to produce sessions that were not overtly prescriptive, yet followed an underlying structure.

> We try to keep it neutral. Sometimes we use references to Christianity, sometimes we use Buddhist techniques. We use meditation in many ways and draw on techniques from a variety of systems and approaches that people find locally in their everyday life, and encourage people to take away things that they find valuable and incorporate into their own lives. We do focusing techniques and all sorts of different breathing techniques – we are teaching people to breathe from the belly rather than from the chest, and we do this particular technique of just watching the flow of breath – so lots and lots of different breathing techniques and relaxation techniques.
>
> (Female group facilitator, occupational therapist)

> ... this [meditation group] is a practical thing, it hasn't got any specific religious or philosophical connections, so you can take it or leave it. If you want to pursue it you can get books and look it up ... they [the organisers] may have religious beliefs, but they don't show it because some people react to that, so you can't take a particular position on that.
>
> (Group member, female, age 55, breast cancer)

Consistently having two facilitators present during sessions was reportedly a significant benefit when dealing with 'trouble'. In the passage on page 109, one of the facilitators describes how the professional backgrounds in health and social care of herself and her partner provided them with organisational tools that might not always be available to organisers of other groups:

> ... I guess from a professional point of view we both do a lot of work. You need to when you do group work or social work. We both have very good training and we both understand the power of groups – the way it can be incredibly positive and destructive as well. We both attend the groups so that there is someone else there if something happens. You know, if something does happen, it just helps if you have two people there – whether someone gets upset and leaves the room, or someone's being domineering. I guess the first problem we had was with a very domineering patient. It really took two of us to get her away ... it was really hard work and we sought help from other people who did group work about how to deal with her ... in the end we found a technique where we were one on either side of her and we had to say 'no, no, stop' and we would put her hands across her chest and stop her. I don't think she was aware of what she was doing and she just wanted to help people, but actually it wasn't helpful at all ... after six months of working with her she calmed down and became a favourite in the group.
>
> (Female group facilitator, social worker)

In common with similarly placed groups in the UK, the meditative process was presented (in both group interactions and in publicity material) simply as a natural and effective means of reducing the damaging side effects of stress, not as a spiritual endeavour. Projection by participants of strong 'new age' or 'alternative' perspectives onto the activities of the group was not actively encouraged – the facilitators feeling that this kind of group image would not only alienate more biomedically minded participants, but might also undermine the credibility of the group within the hospital. Significantly, however, the majority of members interviewed (including the facilitators) openly expressed personal belief systems that were very much in line with holistic and 'alternative' paradigms.

> ... people do develop [spiritually]. You start off knowing nothing and you learn whether you want to or not.
>
> (Group member, female, age 60, breast cancer)

> ... I suppose I think that healing doesn't just come from a pill; there are a lot of other paths to healing, and I think a lot of the things you can do yourself are really good ... I like to think that I'm doing things to help myself.
>
> (Group member, female, age 51, lung cancer)

This issue of personal belief systems (both of the facilitators and members) being essentially hidden during 'official' group activities is significant. In any other type of CAM environment, the open discussion and sharing of perspectives might be a central activity, and one in which members actively engaged. Indeed, it would probably be unusual to find any interest group with a CAM focus (not just in the cancer support field) where this kind of knowledge sharing was not taken as the norm. The fact that our case study group (and others in a similar position relative to the biomedical medical system) attenuates this activity is ironic given that it is possibly closer to 'real' experiences of pain and illness than many individuals who participate in CAM for essentially recreational or 'lifestyle' reasons.

3 Break/debrief

The first meditation or relaxation exercise usually lasted for around half an hour. At the end of this time, the facilitator 'brought back' the group, and individuals were asked how they felt about the experience regardless of whether or not it was beneficial to them. Around ten minutes is allocated to this process. Members are not required to make any comment at this point if they do not wish to do so, but due to the interactional dynamics of the process (with all participants asked in turn), people did report feeling that they should try to make some form of comment, and it was rare to find people refusing to make some remark. Significantly, too, the comments that these 'debriefings' routinely stimulated were almost always either neutral or positive – the researcher observed no occasions when a member made a negative remark or complained about their experience. This contrasted somewhat with what was said in interviews, particularly in relation to the format of the sessions (see below), and perhaps demonstrates the unreliability of user feedback generated in group situations. Some regarded the break (and the 'coming out' of the meditative state which this involved) as being unnecessarily distracting – making it difficult to regain a significant level of relaxation later in the session.

> We've had some absolutely wonderful Zen meditations. It's wonderful, and then you have a break and they want you to talk about it – you want a break but you don't want to talk. I don't like talking about it after.
>
> (Group member, female, age 60, breast cancer)

Others liked the chance to talk about their experiences and give feedback about how they found particular meditative techniques. The facilitators were aware of this problem, but concluded that on balance, allowing people to talk at this point was useful. The fact that the final decision over what format the session should take was with the facilitators is interesting because as we have explored in earlier chapters, many CAM-based groups try to engender essentially egalitarian formats – sometimes going so far as to reject hierarchical organisational structures. While this extreme approach rarely works in practice – the lack of an organising structure usually meaning that a group drifts aimlessly and eventually disintegrates – the fact that it is often at least attempted reflects the underlying complexity of CAM; not limited to the 'medical', its holistic ethos spills over into all aspects of the group dynamic. In the present case study, however, even though there were a number of ways in which CAM influences were apparent, they were not dominant in this key area. 'Power' over the way the group was run and what the group did rested securely with the facilitators.

4 Second meditation

Following the feedback session, another guided meditation was read out by the second facilitator. This usually contrasted with the first one, although again, the group was asked if they had any preferences before it was started. Around 20 to 30 minutes was allowed for this part of the session. The two-part structure was a contentious issue, with members displaying polarised views about the value of the process. Some members reported that the process of switching in and out of deep meditative states was troublesome, while others found that it resonated with them.

> I like the structure and the way they have it in two parts. Actually I think it works quite well – the first part is usually just a relaxing thing so that works well and gets you in the right frame of mind. You are lovely and relaxed and there have been times when I've been so relaxed that I've been really out of it. But it's nice when they ask you for feedback.
>
> (Group member, female, age 51, lung cancer)

> I don't like the idea of having two meditations. I don't know why, but the first meditation is really good and then you have a bad one and it destroys it ...
>
> (Group member, female, age 57, stomach cancer)

In the same way as with the short feedback break after the first meditation, the facilitators took note of the views of members when deciding how activities should be arranged, and addressed this and other issues informally, and through the use of assessment questionnaires which were regularly given to the group. In this case, responses had highlighted that the different idiosyncratic delivery techniques and voices of the facilitators were preferred by different patients. And by extension, this had an effect on the therapeutic benefit that singly guided sessions might provide to any given individual. The fact that formal 'assessment' measures (i.e. questionnaires) were put in place is perhaps an indication of the underlying influence of official healthcare structures on the workings of the group; it may also be a reflection of the professional backgrounds of the facilitators – it being rare to find 'grass-roots' (i.e. groups operating without the constraints of mainstream healthcare systems) engaging in formalised assessment exercises.

5 Group experiential discussion

Following the conclusion of the second meditation, more time was allotted for people to discuss their experiences. Some participants preferred to leave at this point and there were no overt restrictions on them doing so (although, as with any group environment, there may be underlying conventions which make it easier for people to stay and sit a session out, rather than draw attention to themselves and leave). The discussions that took place during this period were generally much looser than in the first break and represent a significant crossover in the overt functioning of the group. Talk ostensively focused on the specifics of members' current cancer experiences, and the meditative exercises. Significantly, however, patients often utilised this time to share CAM-related information (such as aspects of therapeutic diets they were engaged in, or other therapies they were using). This highlights the dual role that this group (and other groups that operate from within biomedical medical settings) can play. While their overt function may be the provision of an 'incorporated' or biomedically sanctioned form of CAM (i.e. meditation), embedded within this can be the facilitation of an interactional arena in which 'alternative' and potentially subversive (in terms of dominant medical paradigms) information is exchanged.

Discussion

In this chapter we have outlined the nature and functioning of an Australian hospital-located cancer support group in which CAM forms a part of provision. As with the case study sites we investigated in the UK, it is useful to differentiate between those located within biomedical structures and those which have developed separately from state sanctioned provision. The case discussed in this chapter falls within the former category. We would argue that the 'semi-formal' location of this group is influential in the way it functions on an everyday level; we also argue that an awareness of organisational context can help us understand the apparent discrepancy between its formal and informal processes.

In this initial Australian case study any expression of 'integration' was at best limited. The group operated in a relatively unsupported and marginalised capacity within a biomedical hospital environment, the CAM services that they provide (or provide information about) needing to be carefully adapted so as not to jeopardise either the continued tolerance of the group within the orthodox setting, or the credibility of the facilitators within their professional roles. Thus, at a formal level, care was taken by those coordinating the group to present a neutral image of activities. And even at an informal level, with 'trusted' contacts, the underlying biomedical backdrop against which the activities of this group were enacted remained firmly at the root of the perspectives that were displayed. The potential philosophical conflict between the meditation on offer and the biomedical core of treatment was glossed over. Interestingly, however, this group was very much like many other groups in the UK study in that, despite the facilitators ostensibly organising things so as not to conflict with the ethos and activities of their host organisation, the group developed an important latent function: it provided an informal arena for interaction, a point for the exchange of ideas and information which went well beyond formal service provision (the content of which would form the basis of any external gauging of approval or disapproval). Participants were shaping and creating aspects of activity within the group to meet their own needs; they attended sessions which, because they took place within the auspices of the hospital, were at least indirectly sanctioned by their doctors and other biomedically situated clinicians. As an adjunct to this, however, they took advantage of the subfunction of the group – that of a social nexus – to facilitate the dissemination of knowledge and ideas which would be very unlikely to meet with the approval of their doctors. Thanks to the existence of a group tolerated within the biomedical system, patients made connections with each other and chatted freely about CAM treatments and processes which they might never otherwise have encountered, and were able to do this in a manner that was not constrained by the same structural influences as acted on the coordinators.

This chapter has been explicitly exploratory in nature. It has focused on a single case study group, but one which, by all indications, is not in an unusual position. The activity observed, and the processes underlying that activity were not remarkable, and participants indicated that the organisation and service provision it represented were likely to be repeated in other similarly placed groups. What the case study has suggested is that in the Australian CAM/cancer support group context, the problems which concern professionals and patients may well share much with those found in UK organisations. Group make-up and activities may seemingly evolve in very similar ways to equivalent CAM-based groups in the UK. The same key issues of legitimisation (of CAM activities), group organisation, group leadership, and the CAM/biomedical tension again emerged, and it is the resolution of these issues which appears to underscore the development and longevity of established groups.

Part 3

Consumption, and perceptions, of traditional, complementary and biomedical cancer treatments in Pakistan

Introduction

In the previous two sections of this book we examined the role of non-biomedical therapeutic practices within the context of UK and Australian cancer care, focusing on such things as: how patient support groups engage with CAMs; the role of evidence in treatment decision making; and the degree to which CAMs challenge or are reconfiguring prevailing understandings of the body and disease. The processes we have identified have been interpreted within a Western sociocultural context; how such processes are played out beyond the West has hitherto remained at the level of conjecture.

In order to begin to fill this gap in our understanding there was a need to conduct empirical, but theoretically informed, research on cancer patients' use and perceptions of non-biomedical cancer treatments in poorer countries. Existing literature suggests that, despite the increasing 'Westernisation' of certain facets of primary healthcare provision in many poorer countries, traditional medicines (TM) still receive considerable grassroots support, particularly in rural or remote locations (WHO 2001). According to the World Health Organization, nearly 80 per cent of the world's population continue to utilise their own traditional systems of medicine despite the increasing presence of biomedical healthcare services in many poorer countries (WHO 2001). Previous research in the area also suggests that people's views of biomedicine in some poorer countries may have been tainted by the failures of certain facets of 'Westernisation' and international development programmes. This has resulted, it has been suggested, in a reaffirmation of the value and importance of traditional practices and beliefs systems (Wayland 2004). However, despite anecdotal evidence of continued support for non-biomedical therapeutic modalities, no empirical data exist regarding patterns of usage of TM and CAM among cancer patients beyond the West. As outlined in Chapter 1, studies of CAM consumption in Western contexts show distinct patterns in usage according to patient characteristics (e.g. gender, socio-economic status and cancer type), yet we know little about potential stratification in access to, and usage of, TM and CAM in poorer, non-Western contexts.

Pakistan represented an exciting opportunity for us to explore some of the issues raised in the first two sections of this book in a vastly different cultural, economic and political context. Offering limited biomedical cancer services, and with a large rural and quite isolated population, anecdotal reports suggested that use of traditional medicine for cancer was high in Pakistan (see Chapter 1 for a more in-depth discussion of the social and cultural context of Pakistan). Whereas the relationship between CAM and biomedicine in the UK has been one of interprofessional conflict and sustained occupational dominance (on the part of biomedicine), the presence of biomedicine in Pakistan is a comparatively recent development, and thus its relationship to traditional modalities was potentially quite different. In many rural areas of Pakistan there exist few or no biomedical cancer services and traditional healers represent the main source of primary healthcare for local communities. In this sense, as opposed to the position of many CAMs in the UK or Australia, TM in Pakistan is in many respects the 'orthodoxy' in healthcare for significant proportions of the population. In this way, its relationship to both the local population and to the state is fundamentally different to that of CAM in the West. Moreover, some traditional modalities in Pakistan, as we shall see in the following chapters, have close ideological links with the state religion (Islam) meaning that such practices may be viewed (and treated) quite differently to CAM in the West. Thus, we decided to set up a research project on TM and CAM in Pakistan in order to extend the gaze of the sociology of CAM beyond the West (see Chapter 2 for an in-depth description of the methodologies used).

In this section of the book (which includes Chapters 7, 8 and 9) we consider data from a range of methodologies to examine how Pakistani cancer patients negotiate this pluralistic and complex therapeutic environment.

The current chapter quantitatively maps out statistical patterns in the consumption of TM, CAM and biomedicine in Lahore, a major urban centre in Pakistan. This statistical data is not as in-depth as the qualitative interview data presented in the following two chapters, but we saw a real need for more generalised contextual data to test the veracity of existing conjecture on patterns of TM and CAM use in Pakistan.

Analysis of the survey data focuses on levels of usage and the influence of age, sex, education and geographical context on use of TM and CAM. Moreover, we examine these patients' perceptions of the effectiveness of different treatment modalities (including different forms of TM) and the relationship between perceptions of effectiveness and levels of satisfaction.

The overall aim of the current chapter is to outline some general trends in Pakistani cancer patients' usage of both TM and CAM, focusing on what practices are being used, by whom, and in what sociogeographic contexts. As seen in the following discussion, the data that emerged from this survey illustrated high levels of traditional medicine use and, in particular, signifi-cant differentiation in these patients' perceptions of certain traditional modalities.

Characteristics of the sample

Before we analyse the results of the survey, it is useful to provide some indi-cation of the sample characteristics (e.g. age, sex, marital status and so on). As suggested in Chapter 2, a total of 362 cancer patients were surveyed. In terms of sex, 41.2 per cent of those who took part in the study were female and 58.8 per cent were male. In terms of marital status, 24.6 per cent of the sample were single, 69.3 per cent married, 0.3 per cent divorced, 5.2 per cent widowed and 0.6 per cent were widowers. Over 73 per cent of the sam-ple earned between 1000 and 6000 rupees per month (between US$17 and $102 per month), which is broadly within the range of the reported national average (see Chapter 1 for more information on the social and cul-tural context of Pakistan). The sample was broadly representative in terms of age, socio-economic status and level of education.

There was also a wide distribution in terms of the range of cancer types. Typically, as we see in Western studies, breast cancer (27.6 per cent $n = 100$) emerged as the most common malignancy. This also appeared typical in that Pakistan has the highest rate of breast cancer of any Asian population (Liede $et\ al.$ 2002). After breast cancer, haematological malignancies (11.6 per cent), throat cancer (9.7 per cent), uterine cancer (8.3 per cent) and can-cer of the abdomen (5.8 per cent) were the most common forms of malignancy in our sample.

Patterns of use of TM, CAM and biomedical cancer treatments

As suggested in Chapter 1, the limited research that has been done on TM and CAM use by cancer patients in Pakistan suggests that, as in the West, use is relatively high. For example, Malik $et\ al.$ (2000) found widespread use of 'unconventional' methods of therapy (54.5 per cent of all cancer patients), with traditional herbal medicines and homeopathy the most com-monly employed methods (70.2 per cent and 64.4 per cent of the sample respectively) (see also Zakar 1998). In this project we sought to measure whether the data from these studies is still accurate (including their applica-bility to different geographic locations), and second, to explore whether there were any patterns in perceptions of, or use of, individual TMs or CAMs. Hitherto no study, including those mentioned previously, had addressed this important issue. Most had been done in Karachi and tended to conflate CAM and TM into a singular category rather than investigating patterns between and within CAM and TM practices. This is despite the fact that research in the West has shown that treating CAM as a singular entity ignores the complexity of how individuals view and relate to particular therapeutic modalities. Thus, we hypothesised that this could also be the case for traditional cancer treatments in Pakistan, and hence our survey was designed to explore these potential complexities.

We found that use of TM and CAM was significantly higher than reported previously, with 84 per cent of all those cancer patients surveyed utilising a TM and/or a CAM. Moreover, 59.7 per cent of the patients surveyed had used more than one type of TM or CAM. In terms of the prevalence of use for particular therapeutic practices, *Dam Darood*, spiritual healing and *Hikmat* (see Chapter 1 for descriptions of the different therapeutic modalities available in Pakistan) emerged as the most commonly used TMs, with use reported at 70.4 per cent, 47.2 per cent and 35 per cent respectively. There was comparatively little use of CAMs such as homeopathy, acupuncture and traditional herbal medicine. The highest rate of use for such practices was for homeopathy with 26 per cent of patients using this modality (31 per cent of all CAM/TM users). Virtually no patients had used other common Western CAM therapies (e.g. nutritional medicine, meditation, reflexology, Ayurvedic medicine or acupuncture).

We were also interested in whether Pakistani cancer patients were utilising a single TM or CAM, or whether they were actively drawing together different therapeutic modalities. By investigating this we would provide some insight into potential commensurability (or lack thereof) between different therapeutic practices, and indeed, clarify the degree to which cancer patients were prepared to try multiple options (and whether this was culturally acceptable) in their attempt to cope with a cancer diagnosis. Were these patients drawing on their traditional beliefs systems (i.e. consulting a *Hakeem*) or were they actively seeking and combining different CAM/TMs?

Our survey showed that, although the largest group of patients used only one TM or CAM (23.8 per cent of the sample), 13.8 per cent used four, 20.4 per cent used three and nearly 18.8 per cent used two. This represents a significant proportion of the sample who were actively combining a range of therapeutic practices within their cancer care. The most common combination was *Dam Darood* and *Hikmat* (use of a *Hakeem*). However, the survey data tells us little about what informs these cancer patients' decisions to utilise multiple treatment options (including traditional and biomedical). Indeed, such a finding raises rather more questions than it actually answers. Hence, in Chapter 8 we unpack patient decision making in rather more detail via our qualitative data generated in a follow-up study to the survey.

The next issue we investigated in the survey analysis was the degree to which sociodemographic factors like age, sex and education were impacting on these cancer patients' decision making about TMs and CAM. Certainly, as outlined in Chapter 1, CAM use in Western countries like the UK and Australia has typically been stratified according to social demographics, with middle-class, younger females representing the 'typical' CAM user. Moreover, there is also research showing stratification according to disease type and disease stage, with, for example, female breast cancer patients reporting high rates of CAM usage (e.g. Morris *et al.* 2000). Thus, we were interested in whether similar patterns existed in the Pakistani context.

The results of this survey highlighted a number of important demographic factors influencing use of TM. The patient's age seemed to mediate use of TM, and in particular, the use of *Dam Darood* and *Hikmat*. Use was highest amongst cancer patients between 11 and 30 years, and then dropped off for older patients. In terms of sex, the results indicated that sex-related stratification (like that seen in consumption of CAM in the West) may be a culturally specific process. Females in our study reported lower levels of TM and CAM use than their male counterparts (81.2 per cent of females versus 86.6 per cent of males), a significant departure from patterns seen in consumption of non-biomedical practices in Western contexts.

A focus of our study was examining whether there was significant differentiation in terms of use or perceptions of specific traditional modalities. It was interesting to note that around 10 per cent more males used *Dam Darood* (76.5 per cent) than females (66.2 per cent) in the sample. Interestingly, sex was not a factor in the use of a *Hakeem* with 35.3 per cent of females using a *Hakeem* versus 37 per cent of males. Once again, this pattern is quite distinct from data collected in Western contexts which has repeatedly shown that females use non-biomedical treatments significantly more than men. In the case of *Dam Darood* – and we expand on this issue in the following two chapters – it is possible that its Islamic basis may influence patterns in consumption. Whereas CAMs in the West have been characterised by some as linked to aestheticism, naturalism, holism and New Age ideologies (which have also been characterised by some as more 'feminine' pursuits), *Dam Darood* remains firmly rooted in traditional Islamic doctrine, perhaps making it more appealing to males (compared with CAM in the West) within this sociocultural context.

Relationships between TM and CAM use and cancer type

As mentioned in Chapter 1, studies have previously indicated that there may be relationships between cancer type and CAM usage (e.g. Morris *et al.* 2000; Salmenpera 2002) and, in particular, significantly higher usage amongst female breast cancer patients. However, as yet there has been no empirical research to tease out the potential relationships between cancer type and TM or CAM use in Pakistan. As it turned out, our data showed no clear stratification in terms of use of TM or CAM by cancer type (Chi^2 = 0.77 [df = 1], p = 0.419), and importantly, when compared with all other cancers, the breast cancer sufferers surveyed here actually had slightly lower levels of TM and CAM usage (85 per cent for 'all other cancers' versus 79 per cent for 'breast'). Bear in mind that males and females were nearly equally represented (males = 57 per cent, females = 43 per cent) in the 'other cancers' category (i.e. the cancer type differentiation, or in this case lack thereof, was not merely a result of a gender split).

This finding is significant considering the clear stratification by cancer type observed in Western contexts (e.g. Morris *et al.* 2000), and as such warrants further investigation. It is possible that, due to lower levels of community advocacy (i.e. compared with the powerful breast cancer lobby in the UK or Australia), breast cancer patients are less likely, due to fewer support programmes, within this sociocultural context, to try all the treatments available, or indeed, to seek out treatment alternatives.

Level of education and use of TM and CAM

Just as CAM use in the West has been linked to higher socio-economic status, it has also been linked to level of education. This is also the case in poorer countries like Pakistan where use of traditional medicines has been speculatively linked to education and socio-economic status. However, no research has been done to assess whether this is actually an accurate portrayal of stratification in local consumption practices. Thus, in this survey we examined the degree to which level of education was a potential mediator of TM and CAM use in Pakistan.

Interestingly, it emerged that there were no clear relationships between general usage of TM and CAM and level of education, suggesting, at least initially, that use of non-biomedical modalities in this sociocultural context cannot be explained by arguments about a patient's (lack of) education. However, when we examined the usage of individual TMs there *was* a distinct relationship. For example, use of a *Hakeem* was closely related to level of education within this sample. The higher the level of education, the less likely patients were to utilise *Hikmat* (see Table 7.1). In Chapters 8 and 9 we draw on these patients' first-hand accounts in an attempt to explain why such stratification exists in use of TM. What emerges is a complex picture of the ways in which use of particular practices is mediated by the desire for social distinction, but also belief in religious ideology.

Are there differences between hospitals?

The hospitals that we recruited patients from were significantly different in terms of their size and population characteristics (see Chapter 2 for further descriptions of the study sites). Thus, in analysing the survey data, we examined potential differences in the use of TM and CAM according to the recruitment site. It emerged that there were statistically significant differences in use of TM and CAM between the hospital sites from which we recruited (Chi^2 = 15.5 [*df* = 3], *p* = 0.01). For example, as seen in Table 7.3,

Table 7.1 CAM/TM use and level of education

Level of education	Non-user	CAM/TM user
No formal education	18.1%	81.9%
Primary school	14.7%	85.3%
Secondary school	16.0%	84.0%
Undergraduate degree	6.3%	93.8%
Postgraduate degree	10.0%	90.0%

Table 7.2 Use of a Hakeem and level of education

Level of education	Non-user	CAM/TM user
No formal education	57.2%	42.2%
Primary	66.2%	33.8%
Secondary	69.6%	30.4%
Undergraduate	81.3%	18.8%
Postgraduate	90.0%	10.0%

of the patients surveyed at Hospital 4, 90.8 per cent ($n = 138$) had used TM or CAM versus 68.3 per cent at Hospital 1 which had the lowest level of TM and CAM usage. It is possible that this pattern relates to the fact that those surveyed at Hospital 4 were on average of a higher socio-economic status (see Table 7.4) to those patients at the other three hospitals, and thus could afford to use a range of therapeutic modalities. However, this is contradicted by the overall data which showed no relationship between socio-economic status and use of TM and CAM. As seen in Chapters 8 and 9, the difficulty with quantification within this social context is that a multitude of factors influence decision making processes, including socio-economic status, religiosity, the need for social distinction, pragmatism and so on. Such complexities emerge strongly in the following two chapters which provide further in-depth insight into stratification in use of TM and sociodemographic factors.

Perceptions of effectiveness of, and satisfaction with, TM, CAM and biomedicine

A key issue in debates about CAM and biomedicine in the West is that of 'effectiveness': what it is, how it is (or should be) measured, and indeed, who should get to decide on such issues. 'Effectiveness' (as assessed by the clinical trial) has been a central concept within the wider evidence-based medicine movement. It has become entrenched in government policy in the UK and Australia (e.g. DoH 2000), despite ambiguity about what it actually means or

Table 7.3 Total CAM/TM use by hospital

	Non-users	Users	Missing
Hospital 1	31.7%	68.3%	
Hospital 2	14.5%	85.5%	
Hospital 3	22.1%	75.6%	2.3%
Hospital 4	9.2%	90.8%	

Table 7.4 Socio-economic status by hospital

	Low	Medium	High	Missing
Hospital 1	75.6%	22.0%	2.4%	
Hospital 2	94.0%	6.0%	0%	
Hospital 3	73.3%	26.7%	0%	
Hospital 4	69.1%	20.4%	7.9%	2.6%

how relevant it is to patients' actual experiences of disease and treatment processes. Within the context of CAM, increasing public support in Western healthcare environments, despite a lack of biomedical 'evidence of effectiveness', has perplexed many within the biomedical community. This has prompted questions about the usefulness of applying biomedical notions of effectiveness and efficacy in contexts where a multitude of factors mediate patients' preferences (above and beyond those related to physiological effect).

In the context of TM/CAM consumption in Pakistan hitherto we had little or no idea how cancer patients viewed TM, CAM or biomedicine in relation to notions of effectiveness. Moreover, we did not know whether these views would be directly (or indirectly) connected with their actual satisfaction with the therapeutic processes under scrutiny. Thus, we decided to ask these cancer patients for their views on the effectiveness of, and their levels of satisfaction with, different therapeutic modalities.

Table 7.5 on page 125 shows these cancer patients' views on the effectiveness of the three most popular TMs in Pakistan: *Hikmat, Dam Darood* and spiritual healing. In terms of the percentage of patients who perceived these therapies to be 'effective' or 'very effective', the figures were: 22 per cent, 57 per cent and 26 per cent respectively. In contrast, we see that perceptions of effectiveness for medical specialists and general practitioners were 94 per cent and 78 per cent respectively. This is a significant differential in perceptions of effectiveness between TM and biomedicine. Furthermore, as seen in Table 7.5, perceptions of the effectiveness of the most commonly used CAM (and virtually the only one used) were similar to perceptions of the most commonly used TMs.

Although perceptions of effectiveness are useful for understanding patients' decision making, and support for, particular therapeutic modalities,

Table 7.5 Perceptions of the effectiveness of TM, CAM and biomedical cancer treatments

How effective?	Hikmat	Dam Darood	Spiritual healing	GP	Medical specialist	Homeopath
Very effective	11%	38%	12%	33%	79%	7%
Effective	11%	19%	14%	45%	15%	16%
Average	20%	16%	19%	14%	4%	21%
Ineffective	17%	14%	15%	5%	1%	20%
Very ineffective	41%	12%	39%	3%	1%	36%
No opinion	0%	1%	0%	1%	0%	1%

we were also interested whether levels of satisfaction would be synonymous with perceptions of effectiveness. Surprisingly, the data (see Table 7.6) illustrated that perceptions of effectiveness are not necessarily related to levels of satisfaction, at least for certain therapeutic modalities. For example, 84 per cent of patients who had used *Dam Darood* reported being 'satisfied' or 'very satisfied' with their treatment, whereas only 57 per cent thought it was actually effective for their cancer. However, in the case of *Hikmat* (*Hakeems*), almost 62 per cent of those patients who saw a *Hakeem* for their cancer reported that they were 'unsatisfied' or 'very unsatisfied' with their treatment. This is similar to the figure of 58 per cent who viewed it as an effective practice (see Table 7.5).

This gap between satisfaction and effectiveness for specific practices like *Dam Darood* is clearly an important issue, and it suggests, among other things, that patients may assess *certain* traditional practices quite differently from biomedical cancer treatments. 'Effectiveness', within the context of some traditional practices, may not adequately capture all elements of the therapeutic process.

In the case of biomedical cancer care, and patients' satisfaction with their medical specialist, there was little difference between perceptions of effectiveness and levels of satisfaction. Rather the specialists scored 96 per cent for satisfaction ('satisfied' or 'very satisfied') and 94 per cent for effectiveness. Homeopathy, the only CAM scored by the patients, received a relatively high percentage in terms of satisfaction (58 per cent), whereas only 24 per cent of the patients who used it actually thought it was an effective means of treating cancer.

The lack of a differential in levels of satisfaction and perceptions of effectiveness for biomedical cancer treatments indicates that some traditional practices may be viewed and assessed quite differently from biomedical cancer treatments. Finding out how patients actually do this, at a grassroots level, necessarily involves documenting the first-hand experiences of individual cancer patients, and hence the development of the qualitative arm of this study discussed in the following two chapters.

Table 7.6 Satisfaction with CAM/TM and biomedical cancer treatments

How satisfied with treatment?	Hakeem	Dam Darood	GP	Medical specialist	Homeopath
Very satisfied	10%	67%	59%	86%	32%
Satisfied	9%	17%	29%	10%	26%
Average	19%	16%	12%	4%	41%
Unsatisfied	59%	0%	0%	0%	1%
Very unsatisfied	3%	0%	0%	0%	0%

Discussion

The aim of this quantitative element of our Pakistan study was twofold. First, we wanted to explore patterns in levels of usage of TM and CAM, and second, patients' perceptions of effectiveness and satisfaction. This would allow us to see whether consumption patterns had changed since previous studies had been completed, and second, to examine, in a generalised way, any differences in how patients view different therapeutic modalities. This, it was hoped, would provide a broad empirical platform that would produce issues of interest to be explored further (and in a more in-depth way) in the qualitative arm of the study.

As it turned out, this quantitative element of the study produced a range of interesting questions which needed further teasing out. On a basic level, the results indicate that TM and CAM usage (at least in Lahore) may be significantly higher than reported previously in the academic literature. It would seem that, either support has been growing for TMs since these studies were completed, or that previous reports under-estimated support amongst local populations. Another previously unknown fact was that a significant proportion of cancer patients are combining different (and often paradigmatically disparate) therapeutic modalities in an attempt to cope with their cancer diagnosis. Previously, we only knew that patients were utilising practices and not the fact that many were actually combining different TMs and CAMs.

This quantitative data also shows us that, just as in the West, consumption of therapeutic modalities is not linear across all patient groups, although, in saying this, the patterns that emerged were significantly different to those reported in studies of cancer patients in Western contexts. Specifically, overall, females used TM and CAM slightly less than males. Although we need more research to tease out this issue, it seems that sex may mediate use of TM and CAM very differently (or be supplanted by cultural and religious belief systems) in Pakistan. Although we elaborate on this further in the following two chapters, it may be that the spiritual underpinnings of some of the TMs available may change the potential intersections of patient characteristics and the use of non-biomedical practices. The fact that there is no strong trend (and that there is in the West) suggests a cultural difference that is vital for understanding wider use and perceptions of particular therapeutic modalities.

It also emerged that there exists little variation in cancer type and consumption of CAMs or TMs. Although Western studies show higher consumption amongst breast cancer patients, in this study breast cancer patients on average used TM and CAM less than patients with other types of cancer. Again, although further research is needed on this issue, it seems possible that both economics and cultural belief may play a role in this difference from the West. As suggested previously in this chapter, due to lower levels of community advocacy in Pakistan (compared with, say, that of the UK), breast cancer patients may have lower levels of access to non-biomedical treatments. Breast cancer advocacy (for women) is so entrenched in Western healthcare contexts that women suffering from the disease generally get exposed to more information and a greater array of treatment options than patients with other malignancies. Moreover, although women with breast cancer (or any other malignancy for that matter) may want to try treatment alternatives, lower levels of wealth in Pakistan compared with those of the UK and Australia may mean that women do not attempt to access these services. In the following two chapters we seek to elaborate on such issues and tease out the potential range of factors which influence treatment decision making.

It is common to see representations of traditional medicine use as a matter of lack of economic capital or indeed one's level of education. Even in Western contexts the scientific community has historically pushed for increased public education to persuade people that scientific development is a positive process. Although more research is needed, these results suggest that education, although a mediating factor, is not linear in its effects. In fact, the only relationship that emerged in relation to education was the *decrease* seen in use of *Hikmat* (*Hakeems*). As discussed in further depth in Chapter 8, use of a *Hakeem* is seen by many cancer patients themselves to be closely tied to one's socio-economic status and level of education, whereas *Dam Darood* was not. Such processes of distinction, as we shall see in the next two chapters, are inextricably tied to culture and religious beliefs systems. Again this illustrates the importance of developing a multi-faceted conceptualisation of traditional medicine and of not conflating all practices into a singular 'TM' entity. These results illustrate the need for studies that are specific to non-Western countries and, furthermore, more research to examine why patterns may differ within such contexts. Such analyses will, clearly, necessitate a focus on the specific sociohistorical context of decision making.

Analysis of these patients' perceptions of TM, CAM and biomedical cancer treatments was also potentially revealing. Although many remained strongly supportive of certain traditional medicines, in the case of particular modalities (e.g. *Dam Darood*), they do not necessarily view them as being effective forms of cancer treatment. However, notions of effectiveness, as conceptualised within a biomedical paradigm (i.e. having a curative function), may be inadequate for capturing the complexity of these cancer patients' views of, and experiences of, traditional medicine. This was particularly evident in the relatively high levels of satisfaction with specific TMs, despite strong views on the ineffectiveness of these very practices.

In fact, it may be that specific TMs (in particular) play a pivotal role in patients' emotional and spiritual wellbeing rather than as potentially curative therapeutic options. This may be particularly the case of TM in Pakistan where healers are often religious figures (as is the case for *Dam Darood*) as well as giving advice and treatment for health issues. In this context biomedical notions of 'effectiveness' or 'efficacy' may not capture the true role and usefulness of such modalities. Moreover, in Pakistan, for many patients, health and faith (Islam) are inextricably linked. Seeking advice and support from a healer may in fact be synonymous with seeking support from a priest or rabbi in a Western context. Being 'effective' at treating one's condition may actually be superseded, in some cases, by a desire for emotional and spiritual wellbeing. Thus, a good outcome might be feeling 'relaxed', 'less anxious' or being 'spiritually balanced', rather than the shrinking of the tumour. This has distinct correlations with dynamics with CAM in the West, where cancer patients often seek different outcomes (some more or less 'concrete') from different therapeutic alternatives.

However, there was not blanket approval of traditional medicines. Rather, stratification in perspectives suggested that different practices are measured using different criteria. *Dam Darood* received considerably more support and much higher levels of perceived effectiveness than *Hikmat,* suggesting considerable variation in attitudes towards different TMs in Pakistan. Although further research is needed to clarify these issues, it may be that a range of different social processes (e.g. religiosity and social status) and individual decision making may be influential in shaping patients' preferences for, and perceptions of, TMs. At the very least these findings demonstrate the need to avoid an oversimplified analysis of the use of TM as a whole and for more research into the differences between therapeutic alternatives.

While our purpose here was to quantify patterns of use, it is important to remember that this study was exploratory rather than definitive. First, the sample is drawn from a geographically specific area, and thus the results can not necessarily be assumed to reflect patterns in other provinces of Pakistan. Second, we only sampled patients from four major hospitals in Lahore, and thus many patients who did not have access to these services (due to economic, geographical or cultural factors) would not be represented in this study. Sixty-seven per cent of the Pakistani population live in rural areas, and it would be reasonable to assume that many people with cancer do not have access to city-based hospitals.

Conclusion

The data we have discussed in this chapter highlights the need to get beyond monolithic categories such as 'traditional medicine' as a whole in order to begin to understand how and why certain indigenous practices are used to a greater extent than others and how the nature of such practices is being modified by the relationship between traditional modalities and biomedicine.

In the context of Pakistan, it seems that perceptions of therapeutic practices are not merely orientated around notions of 'cure' or biomedical notions of 'effectiveness', but rather, support for practices seems more complex and embedded in culturally specific belief systems. However, quantitative data such as that presented above gives us only a limited view of cancer patients' perceptions of particular modalities. Although we can see that there are much higher levels of satisfaction with *Dam Darood* than, for example, *Hakeems,* we still know little about why this may be the case. Moreover, we know little about why in some cases levels of satisfaction remain high, despite perceptions of effectiveness being quite low.

To answer these complex questions and expand on the quantitative data shown here, we designed a qualitative arm to this Pakistan study that would gain first-hand information on why patients are choosing particular treatments and what the implications are for disease and treatment processes. Hence, the following two chapters address these fundamental issues: 1) clarification of factors that drive patients' treatment decision making in cancer care in Pakistan, and 2) how patients experience the relationship between different traditional modalities and biomedicine.

₁tients' negotiation of
₌ ₁erapeutic options

Introduction

In this, the second of three chapters looking at the findings of our research in Pakistan, we move beyond the baseline quantification of action outlined in Chapter 7 to begin to engage with the rather more interesting issue of attempting to make sense of the type of activity identified. Indeed, at this point we shift attention to the sort of questions that have loomed large in the Western-focused sociology of CAM but had previously not been considered either in Pakistan, or indeed in poorer countries more generally. Here, for the first time, we address such questions as: how do patients engage in decision making about the range of therapeutic alternatives? To what extent are decisions grounded in issues of access/cost rather than choice or culture? What influences choice between modalities within the same (albeit artificial) category (e.g. CAM, etc.)? And so on.

Specifically, then, the aim of this chapter is to gain an understanding of how cancer patients in Pakistan negotiate the plurality of therapeutic options (potentially, and, of course, differentially) available to them. As will be seen, we argue that despite the presence of what might be considered to be constraining and even potentially determining structural influences (such as income inequality, the high cost of biomedical treatment and the historically grounded nature of TM), it is important to recognise the active engagement of individuals with the decision making process on a range of temporally and spatially specific dimensions: structural/practical constraint; pragmatic experimentation; and cultural identity and religious affiliation. In so doing we are able to reach beyond over-generalisation and highlight crucial variations of process such as diversity in the utilisation of different forms of TM, and, crucially, the way religion can intersect with, and temper the effects of, processes grounded in status differentiation. It is our contention that an awareness of such complexities is essential if policy promoting the use of TM to address unmet need is to be established in a manner that reflects locally, and regionally, specific priorities.

Conceptual background

Given the lack of previous work in the area, and indeed the lack of directly relevant contemporary sociological work on therapeutic pluralism in cancer care in poorer countries as a whole, it is useful to look at broader work that may contribute to an understanding of the processes discussed in this chapter. Although Western-based, this work identifies certain trends and theoretical ideas that, while needing to be operationalised differently, are worth considering in the context of Pakistan.

However, before doing so, it is worth bearing in mind two aspects of this existing work. First, that interpretations concerning the growth or use of non-biomedical practices are frequently extrapolated from broader theory rather than being CAM-specific. This is evident in, for instance, work on the diversification of healthcare which is couched in terms of: the postmodernisation of the social world (Eastwood 2000); the emergence of reflexive modernisation (Low 2004; Tovey *et al.* 2001); and in terms of new forms of identity work and selfhood (Sointu 2006a; Sointu 2006b). And second, as yet, few of the theoretical assumptions have been challenged empirically.

Perhaps three related elements of this work are potentially most useful for our analysis here. First, that increasing scepticism towards expert knowledge (with what some conceptualise as a postmodern context) is pushing patients away from biomedicine (e.g. Lupton and Tulloch 2002) and towards CAM. Clearly, in the Pakistani context, there are competing sources of expertise for patients to engage with and mediate – both those representing indigenous knowledge and biomedicine.

Second, the increasing utilisation of CAMs by patients has been conceptualised as a product of the limitations of the application of the biomedical model of illness with CAM being viewed as providing a more rounded, patient-centred and holistic approach to illness and disease (e.g. Bishop and Yardley 2004). While country-specific, some of the non-biomedical practices in Pakistan can, in theory at least, be seen to provide this broader approach to healing. While the temporal development of their role may differ from the West, they do, again, in theory at least, share certain points of differentiation from biomedical practices with CAMs in the West.

And third, that use of such modalities has also been viewed as embedded in wider social discontent with scientific developments and technologies (e.g. cloning, stem-cell research), and faith in the superiority of scientific knowledge of disease (e.g. Broom 2002). As a very different world view is often attached to the modalities being used in Pakistan, the potential relevance of this issue is again established.

At an empirical level, research has also shown that treatment choices are mediated by existing forms of social inequality. For example, there is some evidence that decision making with regards to CAM involves considerable differentiation, with factors such as class, gender and geography having an impact on treatment choices. Research has shown that gender mediates decisions to use CAM amongst cancer patients, and that the wealthier middle classes are more likely to access non-biomedical treatments (Thomas *et al.* 2001).

We return to these issues in the discussion to consider whether they hold any potential for understanding the processes of patient decision making in Pakistan.

Patient negotiation of options

The central task to be addressed here then is to begin to understand how individual decision making is being played out by cancer patients in Pakistan in the context of ongoing social change at local, national and global levels. The acknowledgement of the need for research to recognise the condition of an ever-changing (rather than static) environment is well established within many theoretical traditions (Tovey and Adams 2001); it can, as a consequence, become little more than a taken-for-granted assumption that forms the background to research. In this study we were keen to test that assumption by examining the extent to which such change was something that actually constituted a meaningful part of the social context for our participants. The data showed that such change was indeed something more than an abstract contextual development for the cancer patients.

> *P:* I think, for the last 25 to 30 years, there is a major shift from traditional medicines to modern medicines. There is more awareness in our society now about modern medicines. And also, newly discovered diseases are only treated by modern medicines. Traditional healers cannot treat these diseases.
>
> (Female, 36 years, breast cancer)

Another respondent comments:

> *P:* Mostly, people use [the services of] doctors. [In the past] they may have just used traditional medicines, but now the majority goes to doctors ... people do use traditional treatments in our community but I think more people go for modern medicine. I am not satisfied with traditional medicines.
>
> (Male, 17 years, cancer of the bone)

Another respondent comments:

> I: Have there been any changes recently in the way people get access to traditional medicine?
>
> P: *Hakeems*, as we see today, are not experienced as compared to past. As a result they are unable to cure illness. People are now fed up and they need something new. There have been changes in the attitude of people – they seek doctor's treatment as well.
>
> (Male, 37 years, fibre-sarcoma)

Another respondent comments:

> P: People in our community usually go for *Dam Darood* as a first contact. Afterwards, they think of any other method of treatment like allopathic, *Hikmat* ... for the serious disease ... people prefer allopathic treatment. Only proper medical tests can diagnose the disease. Cancer can only be cured by modern medication.
>
> (Female, 19 years, oesophageal cancer)

In these quotations the overriding emphasis is on an evolving legitimacy for biomedicine at the expense of traditional practices and practitioners. The 'power' of biomedicine was a recurrent theme. Participants identified both a trend towards biomedicine and an explicit reason for that trend – its potential impact in dealing with their cancer. However, it is important not to oversimplify what is going on here. Participant perceptions of change were not linear: they were not describing a one-way process towards biomedicine and they were not expressing an uncritical acceptance of what the shift to biomedicine was introducing. Issues raised (to be addressed in detail later) included the tendency of biomedics to 'play God', to 'hit the body too hard', and to be inaccessible to large sections of the population.

> P: I think in future traditional healing would be revived. In future traditional healing would be effective method because people are fed up with modern medicines. Visiting hospitals is a painful exercise, it makes people tired and mad ... medical treatment is costly, while traditional healing is cheaper.
>
> (Female, 30 years, breast cancer)

Another respondent:

> P: I have seen a shift from allopathy to homeopathy. It's good because it's not sharp. It is effective and has lesser side effects.
>
> (Male, 35 years, bowel cancer)

Another respondent:

> P: Traditional medicines have less harmful effects. Modern medicines
> are more harmful.
>
> (Male, 20 years, haematological malignancy)

The situation is clearly rather more complex than a simple move from one
form of medicine to another. The potential for a 'return to TM', although
pure conjecture on the part of the above respondent, is a particularly powerful indicator of the multifaceted and potentially multidirectional
evolution of therapeutic options for cancer patients in Pakistan. But what of
the current situation? How are individuals making personal decisions at the
present time?

On the basis of the evidence from this study, it is our contention that
individuals are actively mediating therapeutic possibilities by drawing on,
and indeed at times being constrained by, personal, social and cultural
resources. We argue that this can be conceptualised by appreciation of individuals' active engagement with three temporally and spatially specific
dimensions: structural/practical constraint; pragmatic experimentation; and
cultural identity and religious affiliation. It is the negotiation (and varying
power) of these dimensions that is crucial to the process.

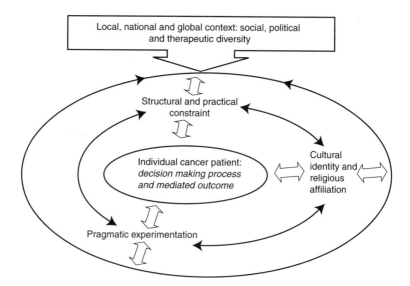

Figure 8.1 Cancer patients' negotiation of therapeutic options in Pakistan. Here we illustrate
how the active decision making of patients is located at the centre of the three
dimensions of influence. These are in turn located within the broader local,
national and global context. The potential for multidimensional impact is noted.

Practical/structural influences
on treatment decision making

In the main, the growth of non-biomedical practices, across the West in general, and in the UK in particular, has occurred in the private sector. Indeed, in the UK their use (with certain exceptions) has had a direct cost implication for the individual, in contrast to core care, which is essentially free at the point of use. As the mainstreaming of CAM has become increasingly advocated so this cost dimension has been recognised as a barrier to use. Moreover (and while a simple causal link is not being argued for), CAM use in the West has remained stubbornly skewed towards the middle classes (Thomas *et al.* 2001).

It is something of a truism, of course, that the context in Pakistan is very different. However, although they inevitably become manifest quite differently at an empirical level, consistencies are identifiable conceptually: the existence of (in theory at least) a pluralistic therapeutic environment; greater cost implications of certain choices over others; a background of economic diversity and so on. The key issue here, therefore, is to examine the context-specific impact of structural factors on decision making. As will be seen, and not surprisingly, evidence from this study highlights quite particular practical pressures underpinning therapeutic choice.

> *I:* Why do people go to *Hakeems?*
> *P:* So far as I am concerned, I think they go to *Hakeems* due to poverty. They can not afford expensive [biomedical] treatment.
> > (Female, 48 years, ovarian cancer)

Another respondent comments:

> *P:* [brother]: Allopathy is expensive while traditional medication is cheap so I think allopathy is better [but] not feasible for everyone.
> *I:* In your community, which type of medicine do poorer people tend to use?
> *P:* Poor people usually try *Desi* medicine first, because allopathic is expensive. People generally try to be cured by cheaper medicines.
> > (Male, 17 years, cancer of the bone)

Another respondent:

> *I:* In your neighbourhood, where do people prefer to go: to a doctor or a *Hakeem?*
> *P:* Most of the people go to doctors; basically it is the matter of money. The wealthy people go to doctors and poor people go to *Hakeems.*
> > (Male, 12 years, diagnosis unclear)

Another respondent:

> P: These quacks are more successful than those qualified doctors. This is because of poverty that people prefer to go to the quack as compared to doctors. Doctors charge 500 rupees and quack charges 25 rupees. There are no ethics, no values, people are bad, very bad.
>
> (Male, 60 years, thyroid cancer)

Another respondent:

> I: Did you travel far for your treatment?
> P: We came from Rajanpur to Lahore.
> I: What is the distance between the two?
> P: Approximately four hundred kilometres.
> I: How much did you pay [for treatment]?
> P: We have spent eight to nine hundred thousand [US$15,000] besides government contributions. We had a business which is finished now and I will struggle until my death.
>
> (Male, 20 years, haematological malignancy)

The issue of cost was not just about receiving the most effective treatment. Rather, it was about the burden of leaving work, travelling to the city, and paying for food and accommodation in the hospitals (see also Nigenda *et al.* 2001).

> I: How do people use different therapies/healers etc.?
> P: Poverty takes them to traditional healers. They are also sensible, and know well that there are specialist doctors for the particular disease, but they are bound to go for traditional healing. People seek the treatments like *Dam Darood,* spiritual healing, as people are poor. They prefer self-medication and traditional healing because they don't have access to modern treatment ... If they seek the help of doctors they have problems with accommodation, food, etc.
>
> (Male, 37 years, fibresarcoma)

While such findings could certainly have been anticipated, at a time when the promotion of traditional practices is being discussed more fully on the international stage, it is important that all assumptions are tested in the field. This is because if cost is essentially the only factor which underpins use of traditional practices (either instead of, or before, biomedicine), serious ethical issues could be raised about the promotion of TM locally, nationally and internationally. However, despite the importance of such constraints, as will now be seen, it is important that we do not oversimplify the situation either in terms of glossing over economic variation within the population or in terms of underplaying other (social and cultural) processes that are potentially central to decision making. We are dealing with a rather more complex situation than an inevitable (and sole) progression towards biomedicine if and when structural limitations can be overcome – one in which the active individual mediation of circumstance remains central.

Pragmatic experimentation and decision making

We define pragmatic experimentation in this context as the willingness and capacity to work through therapeutic options in order to see 'what works'. Of course, it is important to consider such experimentation within the context of the structural constraints discussed above. The capacity to engage in such a strategy varies markedly according to (primarily material) resources, but it is important to recognise that for some it can play a very real part in the experience of having cancer. And while the potential for such experimentation is influenced by context, the form it takes is informed by the nature of social contacts (and therefore the individual's acquired experiential knowledge).

What the data showed was that a number of respondents (with the resources to do so) bypassed or challenged the paradigmatic or ideological bases of the therapeutic modalities on offer, and made decisions purely based on what was going to help them. This could take a number of forms. For some this may entail a willingness to critique the basis of the modality, while for others a 'suspension' of, or removal from, consideration of the broader foundations (albeit possibly temporarily) in pursuit of therapeutic gain was evident. This pragmatism was exemplified by a tendency to try out options, but then to quickly move on if results were not satisfactory.

Such patients are prepared to adopt this approach in relation both to traditional healers and biomedicine. As one young respondent (who it should be noted is talking from the perspective of a social location that permitted access to relatively early biomedical treatment) noted after stressing that 'modern medicine' was his first point of reference:

> P: ... if pain continues and doctor's medicines remain ineffective then people usually move towards *Hakeems*.

Later in the interview:

> P: I think that modern medicines are better. [However,] one can use a knife either to peel an apple or to cut a throat. Similarly science has many advantages and disadvantages.
>
> (Male, 17 years, bone cancer)

There was scepticism amongst a number of the interviewees towards both biomedicine and traditional medicines; this was perpetuated by negative experiences of interactions with, and treatments provided by, doctors and traditional healers. These patients tended to make decisions based on advice from relatives and members of the community, and then, once a treatment had begun, assessed the effectiveness of the practice. As mentioned above, on occasion this occurred without an engagement with the bases of particular practices, whereas at other times it produced a questioning of the logic behind the modality, assessing the rationale behind, and potential benefit they may receive from, healing therapies.

> P: There are a lot of people in our village – most of them are our relatives – who suggested we go to *Hakeems* and *Dam* [so we did]. [The spiritual healer] said that [cancer] was a case of magic.
> I: Who said that it is a case of magic?
> P: [The spiritual healer] said all that rubbish.
> I: Do other people go to this [spiritual healer]?
> P: Yes. When I went to [the spiritual healer] in Lahore, there were a number of people including men, women and children. They came there for different diseases. [The spiritual healer] said, 'Your donkey will die when you get rid of the disease.' I then told him that we can't afford a donkey and above all there is no need to kill any donkey ... they are no good these people.
>
> (Female, 28 years, abdominal cancer)

Cultural/status and religious influences on decision making

We turn now to the cultural and religious. The key point here is to underline how while access to material resources is clearly a powerful factor in decision making, action cannot be reduced to that alone. While (as we will see in our example of an influential cultural process) status aspiration and ascription related to social location action in one domain may reinforce the inequalities of another, we also see when we examine religion how identity and health behaviour are multidimensional.

> I: Have you used [traditional healers]?
> P: My whole family is very educated, my parents, my relatives don't interfere in my matters. I know what is right and what is wrong. I know allopathic is better mode of treatment for a disease like cancer. If I put my ear on views of people then I might adopt some wrong treatment which in turn could worsen the condition. I did not ask any *Hakeem* or quack for help because I feel they are not competent for serious illnesses like cancer. I know we should listen to society and our relatives but I also can't compromise on serious issue like health.
>
> (Female, age unknown, breast cancer)

Another respondent comments:

> *I:* Have you ever gone to a *Hakeem* for any treatment?
> *P:* No, not at all.
> *I:* Why?
> *P:* I don't believe in them.
> *I:* Have you ever gone to a religious healer?
> *P:* No, never.
> *I:* Why?
> *P:* We are educated people ... if you have got a serious disease you'll obviously go to a doctor, not to a ... *Hakeem*. Doctor will examine you and diagnose you, and then you will get proper treatment.
>
> (Female, 41 years, uterine cancer)

Another respondent:

> *I:* What do you think about traditional healing?
> *P:* I think it is better for minor illnesses but not for cancer.
> *I:* Where do people of your locality go for their treatment?
> *P:* The majority of the people here belong to upper class, so they go to specialist doctors even for minor illnesses. They go to the national hospital or doctor's hospital ... There is continuous development in the field of medicine. People believe that it is best for all problems.
>
> (Female, 51 years, uterine cancer)

So how might we begin to understand what's going on here? Well, it is apparent from amongst these respondents' discussion of the type of medicine accessed that each brought with it connotations of status and social standing – the specific traditional medicine being discussed is viewed as the option of the poor and the less educated. It is equated with being in a position that prevents one from choosing 'the best' (see also Nigenda *et al.* 2001), and we might therefore tentatively begin to see this in terms of cultural distinction (Bourdieu 1984) – the utilisation of medicine as a means of underlining social differentiation. Clearly, this is a preliminary understanding of the situation from this initial study, but it is certainly worthy of critical examination in later studies.

Interestingly, however, and in keeping with the sense of complexity that was revealed by the data, such differentiation as is outlined above did not simply constitute a rejection of the local or the traditional in favour of the Western or the global. It was instead a *partial* differentiation that was evident – one based on a separation from only *specific* parts of traditional culture and practice. When traditional medicines were explicitly rooted in religion, specifically in Islam, there was more of a sense of identification with them. On one level, this may appear to induce a potentially contradictory basis for treatment with the combining of *Dam Darood* (which maintains, among other beliefs, Allah's supreme control over one's fate) with biomedical interventions (which seek to intervene in the natural or the pre-ordained). However, the interviews illustrated how many of these patients juggled these seemingly quite different systems of practice, in a complex environment of modernity and intense religiosity. There was a sense that utilising traditional healing like *Dam Darood* was in part about maintaining community solidarity (rather than to differentiate as seen above) and personal faith. What emerged in these patients' accounts was a need to maintain their community identity (i.e. Pakistani and local community identity) and their faith, whilst also maximising clinical outcomes through biomedical cancer treatments. In terms of 'making sense' of such disparate therapeutic modalities, in effect, these patients compartmentalised traditional and biomedical treatments, to ensure the best possible outcome without compromising existing religious and cultural belief systems.

> I: What treatments have you used?
> P: [husband replies]: We did not use any other treatment except seeking help from doctors at [specific hospital]. For her I did not let her use anything other then allopathic. Well, yes she and myself have firm belief in *Dam Darood*. Islam gives you a complete code of life. So being an honest Muslim like others, I have a blind faith in *Dam Darood*. All diseases are caused by God's will, and I think prayer and *Dam Darood* do matter a lot for healing and [we use it] for any particular diseases.
>
> (Female, 47 years, breast cancer)

Another respondent:

> I: Do your religious beliefs affect the way you access traditional medicine /CAM?
> P: Obviously, if we have belief in God. We will certainly do *Dam Darood*. Villagers usually do *Dam Darood*.
>
> (Male, 50 years, throat cancer)

Another respondent:

> I: Do you recite some Quranic verses?
> P: Yes, I do. Being a Muslim it is a duty of every Muslim to have faith in God's knowledge. They really cure illness. If you see in Shaukat Khannam hospital, there will be lots of Quranic verses displayed on walls; and on the entrance desk you can get many of these in photostat papers.
>
> (Male, 56 years, breast cancer)

Another respondent:

> P: The spiritual healer [came] to my home in his car. I arranged a dinner for [him]. He told me to recite a verse for three years, and advised me to keep it strictly confidential and not to even discuss with anyone and after three years I was allowed to tell anyone. I used to recite it daily 1000 times ... It remained quite good and effective for 16 or 17 years ... I feel relaxation in my body after reciting it. In fact I feel I am very closer to Allah. I feel I am the happiest person on the earth. One can't get that much happiness even by spending billions of rupees as I do feel after recitation of those verses.
>
> (Male, 50 years, stomach cancer)

It is seemingly the case that religion is not just an important contextual dimension to decision making but is pivotal to it – intersecting with other structural and cultural influences evident in the process. Identification of the centrality of religion is crucial to making sense of the differentiation in attitudes to various TMs which this chapter has identified.

Discussion

The study reported here was developed as a response to the need for an understanding of the utilisation of the plurality of therapeutic options amongst people with cancer in poorer countries in general and Pakistan in particular. The need for contemporary analysis was underlined by evolving international circumstances. Alongside the spread of biomedical orthodoxy, which became ever more evident throughout the twentieth century, there is now the potential internationalisation of those CAMs widely used in the West. And perhaps most importantly, signs of a shift to a global consensus whereby TM is seen as a potentially powerful tool providing people in poorer countries with local, culturally sensitive means of healthcare. This is seen most visibly in the attention given to the subject by the World Health Organization.

In attempting to make sense of how decisions are made about the range of therapeutic options amongst our sample of cancer patients we have argued that there is a need to take account of three core intersecting processes, their relative significance ultimately being mediated at an individual level.

Not surprisingly given Pakistan's position as one of the world's poorer countries, practical/structural issues were shown to be immensely important in these patients' treatment choices, with cost and proximity to provision emerging as influential factors. An absence of sickness benefits, treatment subsidies, or funded hospital accommodation made it very difficult for significant proportions of the population to seek biomedical cancer treatment.

Although played out in very different ways to the West differential, resource-related access to varying forms of medicine is clearly in evidence here. However, while this inevitably provided a push to those non-biomedical treatments options that were available inexpensively and locally for poorer patients, the results provided very clear confirmation that such decisions should not be *reduced* exclusively to material factors. Decisions about the use, or avoidance, of TMs were also inextricably linked with social context – more specifically with cultural and religious processes.

The importance of religion, and its potential power and capacity to transcend socio-economic circumstances, was seen particularly in the case of *Dam Darood*. Here, traditional medicine could be seen to be addressing important spiritual facets of the disease process – and was often used concurrently with biomedical treatment. Use of spiritual healing and *Dam Darood* was widely seen as consistent with a community's religious beliefs, addressing metaphysical aspects of the disease process (i.e. fear of death/desire for a good afterlife). This sheds some light on why *Dam Darood* received considerably more support (i.e. higher levels of usage; higher perceptions of effectiveness; and higher levels of satisfaction with care) than other traditional modalities in our quantitative work. Support for *Dam Darood* was clearly deeply embedded in wider community beliefs and religious doctrine; aspects that appear to have, for our participants, separated it out from other traditional treatment modalities.

Interestingly, if this part of the data was demonstrating the continuity of belief across respondents, when turning to those practices our quantitative work (see Chapter 7) had shown to be less highly regarded (e.g. *Hakeems*), the converse was evident. Here we saw at least an indication that a process of therapeutic separation was being established. Here those most able to access biomedical treatment were keen to separate themselves from those practices which, for them, performed no function, either therapeutically or culturally. For these study participants this provided a means of status differentiation but one which did not challenge or conflict with the central and powerful dimensions of cultural (religious) solidarity.

Such complexity was also evident in the third core process: the potential for pragmatic experimentation. What was evident here was that any sense of an overly determined notion of the use of particular therapeutic strategies should be avoided. Despite the importance of the above constraints and influences, some participants also reported an approach which focused simply on achieving the best physiological outcome – one which suspended or pragmatically interpreted any ideological assumptions underpinning action. Once again this illustrates the need to avoid assumptions about the outcome of structural and cultural influences at the level of individual decision making – however apparently powerful.

On the basis of our findings in this part of the study we would also argue that there may be some potential in integrating and testing aspects of the theorisation of the use of non-biomedical practices in the West. Albeit becoming manifest in context-specific ways, some participants in this study were demonstrating a clear scepticism towards the claims of a range of 'experts'. And specifically in relation to biomedicine, while patients frequently recognised its potential power in treating cancer, they also expressed the kinds of reservations about it that have been consistently noted in the West – reservations about the harsh, technologically oriented, even de-humanising aspects of the therapeutic process that have been linked to a greater acceptance of CAM. Interestingly, in the Pakistani context there is some suggestion that this parallel process may be underpinning a re-affirmation of the role of indigenous practices, although again this is something that requires further investigation. In short, while the context, historical sequence of events and content of practices are very different from those in richer countries, the presence of biomedical dominance, the awareness of its limitations as well as power and the pluralistic environment suggest that there may be scope for conceptual linkages to be examined in future work.

Given the increased willingness to embrace and even promote 'traditional medicine' at national and international levels, it is crucial that an understanding of such context-specific grassroots engagement with, and assessment of, treatment alternatives is fed into the process. In particular, this study has highlighted the problematic nature of treating TM as a unified category of practices (even within a geographically specific area) – something that would produce an over-generalised, simplistic and distorted appreciation of what is, for these cancer patients in Pakistan, a complex process. Categories of treatment need to be unpacked and the acceptability of their component parts examined in social and cultural context. 'Traditional' and 'acceptable' should not be conflated prior to empirical study examining potential diversity both between modalities and between individuals and social groups.

Chapter 9

Interprofessional conflict and strategic alliance

Introduction

Recent policy statements from global health organisations have emphasised the importance of promoting the traditional healthcare systems operating within poorer countries and promoting further research into the role traditional medicines could play alongside biomedical interventions in addressing the range of health concerns facing their populations (Sphere Project 2004; WHO 2001). Chapters 7 and 8 both re-emphasised this point, illustrating ongoing support amongst local populations for certain traditional therapeutic practices and their relevance to the sociocultural context of Pakistan. However, such arguments about the promotion of traditional therapeutic practices need to be contextualised with an understanding of the specific sociocultural contexts in which practitioners of different modalities are effectively competing for resources, clients and therapeutic legitimacy. Hitherto, there has been no research on the dynamics between traditional healers and biomedical clinicians in poorer countries and the potential conflicts (and alliances) emerging at the interface of traditional belief systems and biomedical healthcare practices (e.g. Nigenda *et al.* 2001). This, it seemed to us, was a major knowledge gap that warranted exploration. What is occurring at the intersections of biomedicine and traditional medicine in poorer countries and what are the implications for various stakeholders?

Chapter 8 explored Pakistani cancer patients' accounts of treatment decision making, their preferences for certain therapeutic processes and how decision making is embedded in particular sociocultural processes. In this chapter, we move beyond cancer patients' perceptions of particular treatment modalities, and towards an analysis of their experiences of the dynamics between different professional groups. In particular, this chapter examines, from the individual cancer patients' perspectives, how traditional medicines (and healers) are viewed by biomedical clinicians and vice versa. This is explored, in part, through their experiences of referral (or lack thereof) between biomedical practitioners and traditional healers. Of specific interest in this chapter is the existence of differentiation in the relationships between *particular* traditional healers and biomedical clinicians in Pakistan.

In a pluralistic health environment like that of Pakistan, interprofessional dynamics are of considerable importance when examining the nature and quality of healthcare services. Just as patient decision making is embedded in religious, cultural and economic factors (as shown in Chapters 7 and 8), so too, it would seem, are dynamics between different professional groups. As we shall see in the following discussion, very specific interprofessional dynamics have developed within this particular pluralistic therapeutic environment which have important implications for patients' experiences of disease and treatment processes. Specifically, conflicts and strategic alignments have developed between biomedicine and traditional medicine as practitioners of different therapeutic modalities compete within a diverse and economically stretched cultural context to provide cancer care. This necessarily extends the arguments developed in the previous two chapters regarding the importance of different religious, cultural and economic factors in mediating patient decision making, to how these very factors in turn influence interprofessional dynamics.

As with the previous two chapters, it emerged that a range of religious and cultural belief systems play a role in mediating the dynamics between traditional healers and biomedical clinicians. It is our contention that the embeddedness of interprofessional dynamics in such a complex mix of factors provides further evidence that simplistic notions of 'effectiveness' or 'economic deprivation' as determining the use and position of traditional medicine and biomedicine cannot (at least alone) explain the various conflicts and alignments between traditional medicine and biomedicine in Pakistan. Once again we see the complexity of intertherapeutic dynamics with religiosity, social status and economic viability each playing a role.

Conceptual background

There has been a significant body of sociological work produced on professional boundary disputes within Western healthcare systems and, in particular, the ways in which specific professional groups seek to establish and maintain a specific position in relation to other actors, and how they utilise particular discursive and practical strategies to prevent others from challenging this position (e.g. Broom 2002; Dew 2000a; Norris 2001; Shuval *et al.* 2002). Such issues have become increasingly important over the last two decades where biomedicine has experienced a relative waning in public support – a waning coinciding with an increasing presence of, and popularity of, CAM (e.g. Eastwood 2000; Lewith *et al.* 2002; Rees *et al.* 2000). In part such developments have been fed by a decreased public trust in, or deference to, scientific knowledge and expertise. The classic case of thalidomide or more recent controversies over Mad Cow Disease have contributed to increased public scepticism towards (but not necessarily rejection of) scientific and thus biomedical expertise. This is not to suggest that there is no longer considerable public support for science. Rather that various societal developments and specific events have led to an increased questioning of the benefits of science and technological development, processes that have in turn been linked to increased consumption of non-biomedical therapeutic practices.

Such processes have perhaps inevitably resulted in ever increasing attempts by a range of stakeholders to reassert occupational control and reconstruct the boundaries between 'evidence-based' medicine and 'non-scientific' medicine. Indeed, the last two decades, and most of the twentieth century, have been characterised by considerable interprofessional conflict and boundary disputes, with particular actors attempting to maintain (or secure) their position within healthcare delivery. The aforementioned developments have also provided the CAM community with increased (albeit tentative) hope for eventual state adoption of their therapeutic practices. To a certain degree boundaries between CAM and biomedicine are increasingly blurred, with some GPs now practising, and/or referring patients to, CAM. Acupuncture, chiropractic and osteopathy are perhaps the most obvious examples of shifting boundaries between what constitutes an 'alternative' versus a 'mainstream' practice. However, despite increased interest in CAM from certain elements of the biomedical community, healthcare (particularly primary care) in Western contexts is largely controlled and delivered by clinicians espousing the biomedical model. Although some cross-sectoral referral is occurring (Berman *et al.* 2002; Coulter *et al.* 2005), communication and intersectoral referral has been, and continues to be, extremely limited. The context of Pakistan, however, is quite different.

Unlike in many Western contexts, where considerable tension has existed between complementary and alternative modalities and the biomedical community (Broom 2002; Chatwin and Tovey 2004), in poorer countries like Pakistan there is some evidence to suggest that intersectoral conflict has not been as binary (Whiteford 1999). Anecdotal evidence suggests that whilst there still remain paradigmatic tensions between traditional and biomedical modalities, some traditional practices may be viewed as valid elements of patient care in their own right. In particular, there is increasing speculation that biomedical clinicians, albeit sporadically, are utilising (or referring patients to) traditional healers in conjunction with standard biomedical interventions. However, there has been no research to examine the veracity of such claims.

It has also been argued that, unlike the dominance of the biomedical view of illness in the West, for people living in rural and remote areas in poorer counties, no single world view is necessarily espoused as superior in all circumstances (e.g. Whiteford 1999). This may, in part, be due to the pluralistic character of healthcare systems in countries like Pakistan, where many patients (and particularly cancer patients) consult traditional healers, biomedics, and even CAM therapists, concurrently (Malik *et al.* 2000). In our research we asked whether this pluralistic historical trend (or lack of ideological hegemony seen in the recent history of Western medicine) would influence the ways in which biomedical clinicians and traditional healers relate to one another.

Despite reports of high levels of therapeutic pluralism in poorer countries like Pakistan, there is also some evidence of difficulty at the interface of traditional medicine and biomedicine (Reissland and Burghart 1989). Some commentators have suggested that practitioners face difficulty in reconciling very different ideological positions (Iwu and Gbodossou 2000), suggesting the potential for conflict and interprofessional gatekeeping tactics. Given the paucity of data available on such issues, we wanted to investigate the nature of interprofessional dynamics in Pakistan and explore how conflicts and alignments were being played out within the context of cancer care.

Referral practices and interprofessional competition

In this study we were particularly interested in how dynamics between professional groups would be influenced by patients attempting to utilise different traditional therapeutic practices and biomedicine cancer services concurrently. Although no research had previously been carried out on this issue, anecdotal evidence suggested that the responses of biomedical clinicians and traditional healers to the use of therapeutic modalities other than their own was not always positive.

Perhaps unsurprisingly, considering the vastly different ideological positionings adhered to and the varying social status held by different clinicians, a significant proportion of patients we interviewed experienced problems, in terms of interpersonal dynamics with clinicians, when attempting to use traditional and biomedical interventions concurrently. It is important to bear in mind that, as illustrated in Chapter 7, a significant proportion of Pakistani cancer patients *do* utilise some form of traditional medicine (around 84 per cent) in combination with biomedical cancer services. The results of this study suggest that this active engagement with different treatment modalities is not unproblematic, with a large proportion of patients reporting significant animosity from their traditional healers and their doctors. Perhaps more importantly, patients reported considerable levels of personal anxiety when having to deal with this interprofessional conflict.

More often than not, their anxiety was orientated around fear of rejection by community-based traditional healers and potential disapproval from the local community. Some patients lived in rural or remote areas in which biomedical treatments were of little historical or cultural significance to the local population (due to a lack of services available). Thus, in some cases, patient use of biomedical cancer services proved a significantly controversial act depending on the reliance of their local community on traditional medicine. This was manifested in such a way that significant numbers of the cancer patients interviewed experienced considerable pressure to conform to the beliefs of elders in their community – people who often had had little exposure to biomedicine and thus had a natural affinity to traditional therapeutic modalities.

A second layer of anxiety emerged in relation to the need for 'being committed' to one practice or the other (traditional or biomedical). It was often suggested that one needed to decide quickly on being supportive of one or the other or risk not receiving effective treatment from either (due to disgruntled clinicians). There were numerous anecdotes of traditional healers responding angrily to the use of biomedical cancer treatments and refusing to continue treatment. Thus, a dominant concern amongst these patients was being disallowed cancer treatment whether it be traditional or biomedical.

> I: Did you tell doctors in [hospital name] that you have used traditional medicine?
>
> P: No, I didn't tell anyone about my previous treatment ... doctors don't consider the patient and never listen properly if you have been involved in traditional medicine. Usually other patients who had practised these healings also don't discuss with doctor ...
>
> I: Did you tell your spiritual healer you had the operation?
>
> P: Well, when I was in hospital, I heard that the [spiritual healer] and [friend's name] were looking for me. After my operation, when I met them, they showed their anger, they were dissatisfied with my decision to get an operation.
>
> (Male, 50 years, intestinal cancer)

From the perspective of the above respondent, and several of the other patients interviewed in this study, the interface between certain traditional and biomedical modalities can be one of conflict, with some healers and doctors attempting to push their patients away from other therapeutic modalities. Whereas doctors were perceived to 'switch off' when patients discussed their use of traditional medicine, discounting many traditional practices, patients reported some traditional healers (particular *Hakeems*) responding angrily to their use of biomedical interventions, sometimes then refusing to treat patients who had accessed biomedical cancer treatments. Such an act was viewed, from the accounts of these patients, as a challenge to the healer's authority, and non-treatment was justified by the argument that 'irreparable damage' had already been done in biomedical treatment. The fact that patients had opted for biomedical cancer treatment was, in turn, used by some of their traditional healers to explain why their particular treatment was not effective.

It also emerged that representations of the 'other' was a crucial method of boundary work and struggle within this pluralistic healthcare environment. Some patients reported traditional healers deploying discourses of 'nature', 'holism' and 'non-invasiveness' as a means of critiquing biomedicine and as justifications for the validity of their traditional practices. These elements were also, in turn, linked to metaphysical elements of traditional practices, including Islamic doctrine, which is seen to transcend the mere physical approach of biomedicine and address their patients' emotional, spiritual and physical needs. Whether *Hakeems* or *Pirs* actually utilise a 'holistic' or 'natural' approach to disease is debateable. Moreover, the degree to which patients actually prioritise such things (nature/holism/religiosity) over scientific rigour or potential cure is not linear (as shown in the previous chapter). However, regardless of the nature of claims being made, it was evident that TM practitioners, much like their CAM counterparts in the West, utilise these discursive practices as a means of professional delineation and bolstering the legitimacy of their practices. Each modality employs particular rhetorical strategies about the 'other' to reinforce the legitimacy of its practices (traditional healers are 'non-evidence based', 'quacks' or 'unregulated'; biomedicine is 'invasive', 'unnatural' or 'harmful'). These discursive practices are part of the process of establishing systems of difference and legitimacy. Moreover, such statements by these practitioners contribute to the generation of attributes – they are involved in the marking of social phenomena as having certain qualities and features (traditional as 'natural' and 'soft' and biomedical as 'artificial' and 'invasive').

The degree to which such discursive practices were actually necessary was inextricably linked to the structural and geographical context within which the practitioner was operating. Biomedicine has very little presence in rural and remote areas of Pakistan and thus such representations have little value where interprofessional competition does not exist. Thus 'boundary work' is necessarily tied to one's need to maintain one's market position. A healer in a remote area may have little resistance to referring to an urban biomedical clinic. A *Hakeem* operating in an urban zone within the general proximity of biomedical services may hold a very different view of interprofessional referral.

The interprofessional dynamics described above, and the discursive and rhetorical strategies of 'difference making', have distinct parallels with interprofessional dynamics between CAM and biomedicine in the West. For years, as outlined in Chapter 1, we have seen various and evolving strategies of exclusion and professional boundary work operating within most sectors of Western healthcare systems. Moreover, lines have been drawn, contested and redrawn around what constitutes validity, how to measure effectiveness and the nature of knowledge of disease. What we see in the Pakistani context is a similar process of discursive delineation as a means of reinforcing or bolstering occupational control of cancer care; however, as we shall see, such practices are not linear across all therapeutic modalities.

In particular, the accounts of these cancer patients were particularly revealing in that they illustrated that interprofessional dynamics were not dichotomous, with considerable differentiation in how particular traditional healers interact with their biomedical counterparts. Moreover, there was considerable stratification in views of, and preparedness to interact with, traditional practices from the medical community. This stratification in interprofessional dynamics, as we shall see below, was often embedded in sociocultural factors rather than a reflection of biomedical notions of 'efficacy' or 'effectiveness'.

Interprofessional conflict and paradigmatic incommensurability

In this study there emerged clear trends in referral practices from traditional healer to doctor. In the previous chapter we saw how the character of the specific therapeutic practices (linked to religious and cultural beliefs systems) influences patient decision making about treatment alternatives. It emerged that similar patterns exist in the referral networks between traditional healers and biomedical clinicians. A dominant theme was that whilst traditional healers like *Hakeems* were highly resistant (and often openly negative) to their patients choosing biomedical cancer treatment, *Pirs* (practitioners of *Dam Darood*) were generally not and had a very different (negotiated) relationship with their biomedical counterparts. We begin with the relationship of *Hakeems* to biomedical clinicians.

It is worth considering at this point the factors that may be influencing the lack of referral between *Hakeems* and biomedical practitioners. What follows is necessarily a preliminary conceptualisation, but drawing on patient interpretations we are able to identify several factors in the general position of *Hakeems* that may have a bearing on the situation. It emerged that there were broadly three factors that seemed to fuel interprofessional dynamics between *Hakeems* and biomedical clinicians. These were: paradigmatic incommensurability, economic competition and historical trends in comparative social status.

First, as seen in the West with CAM and biomedicine, paradigm clashes emerged as central in the mediation of interprofessional dynamics, influencing the development of both conflicts and strategic alliances between traditional healers and biomedical clinicians. Traditional healers like *Hakeems* pursue hugely different views of illness compared with those of biomedical clinicians. In the context of *Hikmat*, the view of illness, disease and appropriate treatment is far removed from the biomedical view of disease. Thus, it was perhaps unsurprising that referral practices between certain traditional practices (like *Hikmat*) and biomedical practitioners were neither frequent nor without problems.

The second factor that emerged as influential in shaping interprofessional dynamics was the desire of individual practitioners to maintain (or increase) their market position in relation to other therapeutic modalities (and even in relation to other practitioners of their own modality). The need to be economically viable in a largely economically deprived sociocultural context shaped practitioners' views of each other. There were noticeable practices of distinction as patients referred to 'real *Hakeems*' or 'those that were not authentic', differences that had clearly been identified by their *Hakeem*. Like CAM therapists in the West, many traditional healers receive little or no funding from the state and are thus effectively competing in an open market environment; this changes interprofessional dynamics from being purely ideological to being shaped by economic necessity.

Third, it was clear that social status was a mediating factor in interprofessional dynamics. *Hakeems,* for example, occupy a relatively low social status in Pakistani society compared with that of biomedical clinicians, and as we shall see below, *Pirs*. The presence of biomedicine is thus potentially a greater threat to *Hakeems* (due to their already limited social status) than it is to other traditional healers.

From the accounts of these patients it would seem that, as a result of such factors, many traditional healers, and particularly *Hakeems,* will not send patients for biomedical cancer treatment. This was considered to be quite a problem for these patients, and in a large part, was seen to be working to the detriment of patient wellbeing. For a number of those interviewed, refusals to refer patients were about the 'stubbornness' of certain traditional healers, rather than a question of the legitimacy or illegitimacy of biomedical treatments.

I: What type of opinion do *Hakeems* have about doctors?

P: *Hakeems* think that what they are doing is a justified and right treatment. Their method of treatment is a lengthy one. They often don't let patients to visit doctors. You know the politics of sellers – for selling their services one always blames others.

(Female, 30 years, breast cancer)

Another respondent:

I: Would a traditional healer refer patients to a doctor?

P: No, these *Hakeems* never refer to doctors. They just want it that, once a patient is with them, they should not go to some other healer or doctor.

(Female, 36 years, breast cancer)

Another respondent:

> I: What do *Hakeems* think of doctors?
> P: They use very strong words for them; both traditional healers and doctors don't like each other. [Our healer] says in our community that both [hospital name] and [another hospital's name] kill people.
> (Female, 35 years, breast cancer)

Another respondent:

> I: What do traditional healers think of modern doctors?
> P: They always say they [themselves] are the best and they have [a] solution for every problem.
> (Female, 51 years, uterine cancer)

Another respondent:

> I: What do *Hakeems* say about doctors?
> P: *Hakeem* [name of *Hakeem*] says that a doctor does not have a treatment for cancer.
> I: What do you think about the *Hakeems* and doctors referring patients to each other?
> P: Both do not refer any patient to each other.
> (Male, 41 years, abdominal cancer)

As illustrated by the above excerpts, *Hakeems* were perceived to be extremely resistant to sending patients to hospitals, and were reported to actively denigrate (and restrict access to) biomedical cancer treatment. For many of these patients, there was a sense that *some* traditional healers were selfish, and perhaps even clinically negligent, in their desire to retain patients. Furthermore, some of these patients suggested that traditional healers may overrate their skills in treating cancer. Thus, overall, professional competition and gatekeeping tactics by traditional healers like *Hakeems* were seen to work to the detriment of cancer care, by preventing timely access to biomedical interventions.

As seen in the second excerpt above, although only mentioned by a minority of the patients interviewed, some traditional healers would also attempt to keep their patients from seeing other traditional healers (sometimes those of the same therapeutic practice). In essence, although lack of cross-referral is certainly ideological in nature (i.e. doctors were seen as particularly problematic, as they represented such a different ideological position), such practices of professional denigration (and gatekeeping) also reflected intraprofessional competition. Ultimately, the desire of some traditional healers to retain their patients will mean that some are resistant to any form of referral, regardless of the therapeutic modality.

As suggested previously, although there seems to be quite a schism between Pakistani traditional healers and biomedical clinicians in general, referral practices were not linear and there exists considerable stratification in terms of referral between specific traditional healers and doctors. The interviews revealed the existence of strategic alliances between doctors and particular traditional practices; alliances which would ultimately allow a compartmentalisation of care, without significant encroachment on the clinicians' respective territories. We now move to a discussion of doctor–healer referral and the case of strategic alliances between particular traditional and biomedical cancer practitioners.

Intersectoral referral and strategic alliances

In the previous chapter we showed how treatment decision making is influenced by a multitude of factors including physiological effect, economics, religion and cultural values. Just as we saw the crucial influence of religious beliefs on patient decision making, religion also played a key role in mediating interprofessional dynamics and referral processes between doctors and traditional healers. We saw in the discussion above that biomedical clinicians largely ignore *Hikmat,* and in turn, *Hakeems* generally do not refer to doctors. However, in the case of *Pirs* there emerged a strategic alliance between the traditional and the biomedical that was forged on common paradigmatic values – Islam. This finding reflects the analysis presented in Chapters 7 and 8 which illustrated the centrality of religious values in patients' decision making about traditional medicines (and their preference for *Dam Darood*). Similarly, their healers' views of doctors (and vice versa) were inextricably tied to religious values. It is here that the Pakistani situation departs from that of the West where CAM therapists and doctors often have very little in the way of shared values. In a cultural context where Islam transcends everyday practice (even healthcare practices), a religious commonality can create important linkages regardless of views regarding clinical 'effectiveness' or 'treatment efficacy'. The social status of *Pirs* or practitioners of *Dam Darood* as important Islamic figureheads fundamentally alters their relationship to biomedical clinicians.

As we can see from the excerpts presented below, according to the majority of the patients interviewed, their doctors would not refer them or other patients to *most* traditional healers. The exception, as seen in the last excerpt, was *Dam Darood.*

I: What do doctors think of traditional healing?
P: They don't believe in traditional healing as there is no clinical proof.

I: Do [doctors] refer patients to traditional healers?
P: No, never. They say that traditional healers are quacks.

(Female, 51 years, uterine cancer)

Another respondent:

P: Doctors don't refer to traditional healers ... doctors don't believe in traditional medicine. [They say] traditional healers play with the lives of people.
I: Would a modern doctor refer a patient to a traditional healer?
P: No, they don't refer.
I: What is the reason?
P: They say their treatment [biomedical treatment] is appropriate.

(Male, 50 years, throat cancer)

Another respondent:

I: Do traditional healers refer patients to doctors and doctors refer patients to these traditional healers?
P: Traditional healers usually don't refer patients to doctors ... Doctors suggest *Dam* but they don't refer them to [other] traditional healers.

(Female, 48 years, breast cancer)

As seen above in the first two excerpts, and in the majority of these patients' accounts, there is significant negativity from doctors towards traditional medicines in Pakistan, with most of their doctors refusing to refer to traditional healers. The one exception was *Dam Darood* – an exception that featured in a number of the patient interviews. *Dam Darood* was viewed by the majority of these patients' doctors as suitable as a complement to biomedical treatments based on a number of crucial factors. First, *Dam Darood* is a practice deeply embedded in Islamic ideology – an ideology pervasive in Pakistani society, even within the so-called scientific institutions like the cancer hospitals we recruited from. The Quran would often be quoted by doctors and Quranic sayings placed on the walls of the cancer wards. Second, *Dam Darood* was perceived to pose less of a threat to medical expertise due to its religious base and metaphysical rather than physiological ambitions (i.e. seeking assistance from Allah rather than intervening through drugs or surgery (see the first patient quote on page 140).

According to a number of patients interviewed, doctors would be more than happy to refer patients for *Dam*, potentially, it would seem, because it posed no real threat to their position within the healthcare system – it merely functioned as complementary to these patients' biomedical and physiologically focused treatment. Moreover, culturally, in Pakistan, the Quran is used as a guide for all decisions in life (even doctors would use phrases in clinics like 'Allah willing') and thus utilising *Dam Darood* whilst undergoing bio-medical care is a wholly 'natural' therapeutic combination in this cultural context.

Interestingly, *Pirs* (practitioners of *Dam Darood*) would also promote use of biomedical cancer treatment in combination with their own prac-tices. Several patients were told explicitly by their healer that they must use *Dam Darood* alongside biomedical cancer treatment. Thus, we see an infor-mal process of cross-sectoral association. This relationship can be seen as both an ideological and strategic alliance in a context where shared values which transcend the physiological allow modalities to work together. With fewer competing interests than, say, those of doctors and *Hakeems, Pirs* and doctors are able to refer their patients to each other whilst also maintaining their legitimacy and relative social status.

The patients themselves often pointed out the differentiation between the traditional healers in terms of their approach to, and support for, biomed-ical cancer care. There were numerous anecdotes of *Hakeems* being resistant to referral and *Pirs* or spiritual healers as directing patients towards biomedical care whilst continuing their treatment as well.

I: What do [*Hakeems*] think of modern doctors?
P: They say doctors' medicines are not too good. If you use it for one purpose it causes many other side effects, and curing of one disease leads to some other disease, like curing of temper-ature causes bad stomach-ache.
I: So, [*Hakeems*] think that doctor's medicine is ineffective because it has side effects.
P: Oh yes.
I: And what is the opinion of spiritual healers [*Dam Darood*] about doctors?
P: They advise to consult doctors. They say along with *Dam* use the services of doctors.
Brother: They say physical and spiritual healing should be used side by side.

(Male, 17 years, bone cancer)

The above excerpts illustrate an interesting differentiation between the perspectives of *Hakeems* and *Pirs*. Whilst the *Hakeems* view themselves as an autonomous healer, treating the 'whole' person, the spiritual healers or *Pirs* view their practices as working with the biomedical treatments, and have developed a mutual process whereby each are prepared to allow patients to be treated by each other. The acceptability of *Dam Darood* seems to be closely linked with the importance of Islam in most segments of Pakistani society, including the medical establishment. Drawing on the 'divine' to assist the emotional and physiological wellbeing of the patient does not seem to be perceived to interfere with the biomedical treatment process. However, in the case of *Hikmat,* which presents itself as a largely autonomous modality for treating disease, the relationship between the 'traditional' and the biomedical is much more complicated, with conflicting ideologies, resulting in, as we have seen, interprofessional conflict and gatekeeping tactics.

Discussion

Within a pluralistic therapeutic environment like that of Pakistan, interprofessional dynamics have very real implications for patient care. Previous research has shown that biomedical clinicians' approaches to alternative therapeutic modalities are varied (Hsiao *et al.* 2006) and have very real implications for both the client–practitioner relationship and the quality of care given to the patient. Likewise, gaining an understanding of the complex relationships between different traditional and biomedical therapeutic modalities is crucial for improving the care given to cancer patients in Pakistan.

From the data gathered in this study we can see that there are a multitude of factors that are influencing interprofessional dynamics within the Pakistani context. Clearly, some practitioners of different modalities are engaging in forms of boundary work and utilising a range of professional gatekeeping tactics (be they practical or discursive) as a means of gaining or reinforcing occupational dominance (or their current positioning) within this therapeutic environment. As we have also seen in the West, practitioners utilise discursive and rhetorical strategies as a means of maintaining their own legitimacy and contesting that of the 'other'. Moreover, some practitioners in this context (both biomedical and traditional) seem to be utilising explicit strategies (i.e. non-referral) to retain direct control over patient care. The general lack of intersectoral referral, from these patients' perspectives, was a major problem in accessing effective and timely cancer care. In certain cases, patients had delayed seeking biomedical help (to the detriment of their health) due to what they perceived to be inappropriate advice from their traditional healer.

The relationship between *Hakeems* and the biomedical community in Pakistan emerged as particularly problematic, with both the healers and doctors refusing to refer to each other. As suggested above, the basis of these dynamics seemed to rest on three important factors: paradigmatic incommensurability, economic competition and historical trends in comparative social status. This combination of factors seemed to make it almost virtually impossible for these clinicians to refer to one another and in many cases resulted in highly unsatisfactory levels of care. The attitude of doctors to traditional healers like *Hakeems* was also perceived to be highly problematic for patients who were seeking to utilise different therapeutic practices. Doctors were represented as largely writing off traditional practices and refusing to engage with patients over their use of such practices or engage in dialogue over their validity.

A final key finding for this chapter was the apparent strategic alliance forged between *Pirs* (those practitioners of *Dam Darood*) and doctors. As shown above, both doctors and *Pirs* would refer to each other and actively encouraged the use of each other's practices. It would seem, from these patients' accounts, that this reciprocity is embedded in both religiosity and the metaphysical focus (both of which are connected) of *Dam Darood*. Unlike the animosity seen between *Hakeems* and doctors, there was acceptance of the need to combine *Dam Darood* and biomedical cancer care – an acknowledgement that seemed to be based on the Islamic foundations of these particular traditional practices. Within this relationship there seemed to be a strategic compartmentalisation of practices – *Pirs* deal with the metaphysical and doctors with the physical, a process that is functional in the sense that the territory (and roles) of particular modalities are clear and not overlapping. These patients' accounts suggest that doctors maintain a high degree of respect for the Islamic basis of *Dam* and view *Pirs* as different but complementary to biomedical cancer care. Thus we see stratification and strategic reciprocation in the interprofessional dynamics between traditional medicine and biomedicine in Pakistan.

This finding is particularly important, in that it illustrates the importance of reflecting the complexity of the interface of traditional medicine and biomedicine in poorer countries. As seen here, different therapeutic modalities may have very different views of – and interact very differently with – biomedical clinicians and organisations. Clearly, such relationships are shaped, as seen in the data presented here, by different social and cultural processes and institutions (e.g. religion).

Conclusion

At the outset of the book we outlined our approach to researching CAM and cancer; we also set out what the book was intended to provide, and, indeed, what it wasn't. We located the work within both its social and its academic contexts. It is worth beginning this concluding chapter with a re-statement and development of that position. Having done so, we will draw out what we consider to be the key themes to have been identified and developed during the research – first from the UK and Australia, second from the studies in Pakistan and third when looking at the data as a totality. Given the relatively undeveloped nature of research in this area we will round off both the chapter and the book with some immediate priorities for social research into non-biomedical practices and cancer care in both richer and poorer countries.

As a first point of reference it is important to reinforce the point that what has been conducted and written about is a piece of *social* research. With so much attention being focused on the generation of 'evidence', we see our work as standing alongside, but distinct from, that emphasis. Our agenda is concerned with how individuals, and groups of people, engage with, and mediate the plurality of therapeutic options in the context of their own lives and the social setting within which those lives are led. Again, as we noted earlier, this is work which may well in time inform policy making – the generation of 'evidence' in itself will have little utility without a broader appreciation of the motivations and processes underlying the actions of practitioners and consumers. However, our approach is grounded in the belief that a premature focus on the need for immediate policy outcomes delimits the nature of questions being asked and therefore the understanding generated. At this stage, the pursuit of policy 'solutions' should not be the driving force behind research.

It is also worth clarifying how the studies are located within this social, rather than medical, research agenda. This is perhaps more straightforward for the work in the UK and Australia than Pakistan. The work in the richer countries is located within the broader sociological study of the use and provision of CAM. Specifically, our aim was to broaden out the agenda to consider group-based, rather than individually focused, action. And, while recognising that the term 'sociology of CAM' represents a loose rather than rigid research framework, the conceptualisation of the study is relatively unproblematic. The situation with the study of Pakistan is slightly more complicated. Given the lack of research in that country on social aspects of cancer, TM use and so on, there was no obvious conceptual framework within which to operate. Clearly, there is a long history of anthropological research in Asia as in other parts of the world, but little of explicit and immediate relevance. As such, our approach was to keep data collection as unstructured as possible while considering the relevance, at a conceptual level, of insights from the sociological study of non-biomedical practices in richer countries. With an ever-changing global environment, we consider it important that the study of the intersection of CAM, TM and biomedicine should start with as few preconceptions as possible. This approach, and the focus on one-to-one interviews, inevitably (as with all methodological decisions) impacted on the nature of data generated. We consider our analysis to be neither total nor complete. And as we will return to later, there is a substantial research agenda still to be engaged with.

The research in each of the countries should therefore be treated as the first stage of a long process. Each can be seen as opening up new lines of enquiry to some extent. It is also important to avoid seeking out inappropriate links between data from the different settings where they do not exist simply on the basis of a seemingly shared core focus. The settings are very different, as are the research questions needing answers at this stage and the approaches needed to answer them. Having said that, interesting, and potentially useful, linkages at a conceptual level (one step removed from the empirical) can be identified. These though should be treated as the basis for further study and not as definitive in their own right.

We move now to the development of knowledge that can be drawn from our research in the UK (and Australia). It will be recalled that the academic starting point for the study was that although there was anecdotal evidence that CAM was being accessed through patient support groups, we actually had little or no understanding of the nature of those groups, the way in which their structural location impacted on their form and functioning and, crucially, the extent to which they are offering anything innovative for their participants. So we needed to ask whether, and to what extent, the presence of support groups provides a forum for the enactment of therapeutic processes which are both fundamentally distinct from, and indeed challenging to, the core biomedical provision? In gaining insight into this and related questions we can begin to assess how such groups are placed within the totality of provision.

Once engaging with the nature of the history and evolution of such groups, the importance of location and/or affiliation became readily apparent. More specifically, the tension between structural position and the enactment of therapeutic processes emerged as pivotal to the provision of CAM. It was this matter of physical location (and/or organisational interdependency) that underpinned the core differentiation between Type 1 and Type 2 groups. Regardless of group type, however, a sensitivity to what was being offered was evident in all groups and the need to retain group viability evident, although this manifested itself in different ways according to the group. Typically, in NHS-affiliated groups it was reflected in a playing down of the esoteric and 'different' nature of what was being offered and a delimiting of provision to that that was deemed to be less threatening. And while independence allowed Type 2 groups to be more overtly 'CAM-centred', the survival imperative was also seen to influence action there. This underlying pressure, reflecting an awareness of marginal status and limited power, necessarily impacted on the functioning of groups at all sorts of levels and this in turn, of course, impacted both on what was available to participants and on their experience of that. At times, this produced fascinating informal processes such as those seen in our case study in Australia where participants radicalised the opportunity presented by the group to push the boundaries of therapeutic options, but only outside of the formal physical confines of the group.

This tension between the potential to offer something challenging and innovative and the survival imperative of the groups is absolutely central to understanding the extent to which innovation or challenge is possible within these groups; it led us to the identification of 'confined innovation' as a way of conceptualising what is going on. There is no doubt that innovative practices are being established – practices that allow, for instance, access to forms of therapy that may otherwise fail to be used by patients. Indeed, in many cases the groups provide an introduction to non-biomedical practices. But if the 'CAM project' is to be understood as providing something more than merely a peripheral adjunct to core provision, then boundaries must inevitably be challenged and the extent to which this is currently the case is very much open to question. While the range of therapies that are theoretically open to support groups to provide information on and advocate is extensive, in practice, through filtering processes by those with a stake in running and ensuring the long-term viability of the group, these are delimited to the least threatening to biomedicine. The 'constraint', therefore, is frequently self-imposed, but imposed through an awareness of the dangers of pursuing an overly radical agenda. At times, for instance, both publicly displayed literature and publicly enacted sessions stand in sharp distinction to deeply held beliefs about more challenging biomedical practices.

When trying to make sense of the role and impact of support groups in the provision or advocacy of CAM, it is important to see processes as multidimensional. What is available to patients cannot be reduced to what key figures in the groups would ideally like to offer, and indeed the functions of the groups cannot be reduced to what is formally available. Operating within the confines of a marginal status and a vulnerability to external critical assessment, strategies are adopted which not only serve to place what is offered within set limits but which also then facilitate the development of informal processes – be these interactions between organisers and participants outside of the formal meetings, or indeed between participants themselves similarly beyond the physical limits of the group sessions.

Like the UK and Australian data, the data emerging from the Pakistan research was necessarily a preliminary look at processes occurring at a grassroots level in this unique sociocultural context. It was, as we have emphasised, the first study of its kind in Lahore and sought to provide a platform for further research into cancer care in Pakistan. Given the fact that biomedical cancer research is virtually non-existent in Pakistan it is perhaps unsurprising that the data we presented provides unique insight into a variety of complex social processes occurring at the point of healthcare delivery.

On the face of it, our quantitative work illustrated extremely high levels of use of TM amongst the population surveyed, seemingly reinforcing anecdotal evidence and some previous work suggesting that TM is playing an important role in cancer care in Pakistan. It would seem initially that use of TM (in combination with biomedical cancer care) is in fact the norm rather than an atypical approach to cancer treatment. However, the complexity of consumption practices was also evident in the data with considerable differentiation in these patients' perceptions of different traditional therapeutics. It quickly became clear that examining TM as a singular, linear entity does not accurately reflect the grassroots experiences of patients. This point is pivotal to our understanding of patients' use and perceptions of TM for cancer care in Pakistan. Although we knew traditional practices maintained an ongoing presence in Pakistan, we did not know that patient perceptions varied considerably depending on the nature of the practice; this, it would seem, correlates with observations of CAM consumption in the West showing considerable differentiation according to the specific treatment modality as well as individual patient biography. The data showed fascinating 'inconsistencies' in patient perceptions of TM. Many patients, it would seem, consider *Dam Darood* to be largely 'ineffective' but are largely satisfied with this traditional practice, throwing doubt on the relevance of Western conceptions of 'efficacy' and 'effectiveness' as informing decision making regarding TM in this cultural context. This is quite crucial in terms of the development of policy driving the incorporation of traditional practices into the healthcare systems of poorer countries like Pakistan. However, we needed to know more about why this differential existed. In talking to individual patients about their experiences of making treatment decisions we found that preferences for traditional medicines varied in relation to the paradigmatic basis of the therapeutic practice and the social standing of the practitioners. When teased out in the context of individual interviews it became clear that various sociocultural processes were occurring which were central to the mediation of patient decision making and interprofessional dynamics (and thus, quality of care).

Complexity rather than simplicity pervaded patient accounts of their engagement with therapeutic options. A range of influences were in evidence and the impact of each was inextricably tied to the particular biography of the individual cancer patient. It has been previously suggested that use of traditional practices is at least in part related to economic deprivation and lack of access to biomedical services in poorer countries. However, it would seem from our work that this is a rather simplistic representation of patients' engagement with different therapeutic options, and that in fact, patient decision making is influenced by a range of factors including: structural and practical constraint; pragmatic experimentation; and cultural and religious affiliation. Each of these factors seems to play a mediating role (albeit at differing levels of significance) for all cancer patients, and thus decision making must be seen as a multifaceted and non-linear process that is culturally specific. Our data is of course shaped by the nature of the approach we took to data collection, that of individual patient interviews. This enabled a close examination of individual concerns and experiences rather than, say, observation of group or community behaviour in relation to healthcare. Much anthropological work has taken the latter approach and thus has provided a valuable but different perspective on such processes. For us, individual interviews provided a specific form of access to patients' experiences.

The role of cultural belief and, in particular, religious belief systems, emerged as quintessential in the shaping of the dynamics between practitioners of different therapeutic modalities. The relationships between biomedicine and traditional modalities, it would seem, are inextricably linked to paradigmatic commensurability and social status, rather than solely simplistic notions of treatment 'effectiveness' or 'efficacy'. In fact, it appears that cultural beliefs and religious values play an incredibly strong role in shaping the structure of (and alliances within) the Pakistani cancer services. Whereas Western healthcare systems are heavily influenced by notions of 'evidence' and 'evidence-based practice', within this social context shared religiosity and compatible therapeutic objectives (i.e. healer addresses spirituality and doctor addresses physiology) enable at least a partial melding of 'the traditional' and 'the modern'.

This differentiation between different traditional practices (both in terms of patient perception and interprofessional dynamics) has important implications for global health policy espousing the promotion of traditional health practices. Any such policy trajectories must acknowledge complexity at the interface of traditional medicine and biomedicine in Pakistan, and the varying ways in which patients relate to different treatment modalities. A blanket espousal of the promotion of 'the traditional' ignores the complexity of interactions and experiences at the grassroots level.

Conceptual parallels

Bearing in mind the earlier stated proviso about the need to be wary of establishing artificial parallels, a number of theoretical links can be identified between the Pakistan data and that retrieved from the UK and Australia. First, each of these studies was informed by the notion of a high status professional group (i.e. biomedicine) versus a peripheral (CAM) or economically restricted (TM) therapeutic alternatives. In the case of both CAM and TM, their position tends to be weak in relation to biomedicine and thus patients' experiences (and practitioners' dialogue with their patients) are in many ways shaped by this dynamic. Both in the Western contexts and in Pakistan we saw how practitioners and patients attempt to negotiate this complex landscape. For the patients, the act of drawing on a multiple of therapeutic alternatives tended to be about using all the potentially 'effective' options available without such practices working to the detriment of their overall wellbeing (such as creating animosity between their traditional and biomedical practitioners). For practitioners, their concern seemed to be centred on whether to create alignments, 'go it alone' or contest the legitimacy of the other (i.e. biomedicine). In both the cases of CAM and TM, therapeutic practices (whether biomedical, traditional or CAM) were shaped by an awareness of power dynamics and ideological dominance.

However, theoretically, the relationship between traditional medicine and biomedicine is complicated by the tendency of the metaphysical to transcend the physical in the context of Pakistan. Religiosity creates a point of connection between the 'modern' and the 'traditional', linking potentially disparate therapeutic approaches through common metaphysical objectives – to maintain one's faith and religiosity in disease and treatment processes. Thus, as opposed to the secularised, individualised Western subject, in the Pakistani context, collective values were seen to function to bring together potentially competing interests for a mutual cause.

There is nonetheless a need for a focus on how Western processes of individualisation may be contributing to the evolution of patient experience and decision making in such contexts. Whilst, as suggested above, collective values seem to have a strong influence on decision making, it was also evident that patients were negotiating a multitude of influences that cannot be reduced to those imposed by the collective. In fact, it may be theorised that as increasing numbers of therapeutic options are made available in contexts such as Pakistan, individual decision making may become increasingly driven by individualised goals rather than collective values.

What of the role of science and evidence in each of these social contexts? It seems clear that, although religiosity plays a strong role in Pakistan, in all three contexts examined here, there was awareness of the potency of scientific technologies in the treatment of disease. However, in each of these contexts significant numbers of individuals (or group members) also expressed doubt about inherent superiority of biomedical models of disease treatment. In the Western contexts, doubts about science tended to be centred on the limitations of scientific measures and technologies (particularly their limited physiological scope), whereas in Pakistan, doubts about science tended to be expressed in the context of the power of Allah and the potentially transcendental nature of disease. Faith in science is thus mediated by the power of competing ideologies. Thus it would seem that TMs embracing prevailing religious values occupy a different, and potentially more powerful, position than, say, CAM therapists in the West.

Looking ahead

So what are the next stages in the sociological study of the use of non-biomedical therapies in cancer care? Given the underresearched nature of the area both in richer and in poorer countries, the agenda is substantial. In richer countries it could be argued that studies grouped into four main themes are needed to extend analysis to the 'next level'. These are research based around professionals and providers; patients; organisations; and that focused around international comparison. The following provides brief examples of the kind of work that is now required. It is, of course, meant to be illustrative rather than definitive.

Issues surrounding professional authority over the provision of treatment for cancer patients remain pivotal to an understanding of the area. As we have seen throughout this book, patient engagement with CAM (in this case via support groups) remains heavily influenced not only by the actions of biomedical practitioners, but crucially, by the perceptions and expectations of others about the power and influence of these practitioners. Elsewhere (Broom and Tovey forthcoming) we have begun to look at this in more detail, considering not only differences within medicine but also the potential mediating influence of nurses in cancer patients' experience of accessing CAM. While we have existing research outlining attitudes amongst biomedical practitioners, we need much more in-depth knowledge of their actual practices and how they interrelate and shape the development of professional action. Such work needs to be based around a fundamental acknowledgement of professional interconnectedness and the subtle nuances of power and authority.

For the next phase of work with patients there is a need to reach beyond the broad category of the 'cancer patient' to explore the differing processes surrounding people in very different circumstances. As we saw in this research, people engage with support groups in different ways depending on disease stage. We need much more focused work to address this issue of disease stage in more detail as well as a range of other variables such as type of cancer.

Our work with support groups is one example of how a focus on organisations can provide a fresh angle to research in the area. Work based on organisational case studies in particular provides a means of bringing together many outstanding concerns in order to explore them in a single context. As mentioned above, CAM/cancer research now needs to move beyond the simplistic identification and quantification or description of attitudes amongst participants. What is needed is an understanding of how action is created and played out in real-life contexts. Work engaging at the level of individual organisations facilitates a focus on patients as well as the various professionals and other stakeholders who have an influence on patients' care (e.g. managers and policy makers). Moreover, the different levels of organisational functioning can be examined via a range of methods including microlevel techniques such as conversation analysis as well as broader ethnographic approaches. The varying influence of specific organisational doctrines should be central to analyses.

The fourth grouping, comparative analysis, reflects the fundamentally international nature of the sociological agenda rather than a more parochial policy-based one. Issues to be addressed within a sociology of CAM (and cancer) do not exist in geographical isolation. Many of the questions to be answered are similar across richer countries. However, because of structural and cultural differences between those countries there is an opportunity to unpack some of those issues. The varying proportions of public, as opposed to private, mainstream provision of cancer care is one example of how diversity is evident across richer countries. This in turn impacts on the consumption of health practices. There is considerable potential to enhance understanding through comparative work across international boundaries.

We now turn to the next steps for social (and sociological) research on TM and CAM in Pakistan and, indeed, issues related to traditional medicines in other poorer countries. On a broad level we argue that there is merit in further exploring if, and how, the findings and foci of the Western sociology of CAM can be extended and tested elsewhere. This work can bring a fresh perspective to an area hitherto dominated by anthropology. The reason for this is that there has been much work done involving observation and examining grassroots processes at the level of culture, but little addressing questions like those raised here, such as what constitutes 'effectiveness' and 'efficacy', and how such notions are viewed within different social contexts. Much as been written about both public perceptions of science and scientific developments in the West, and about declining popular belief in scientific expertise. This has, in turn, been linked to wider societal changes such as increased individualism and the so-called postmodernisation of everyday life. These processes, it has been argued, have been accompanied by increased distrust in biomedicine and support for CAM. However, we still know little about public perceptions of science and scientific knowledge in poorer countries. How do people view science and scientific expertise in sociocultural contexts where religious ideology is omnipresent? How does belief in the transcendental alter public perceptions of knowledge of physiology? Such questions will inform further investigation into what shapes conflicts and alignments between and within TM and biomedicine in poorer countries like Pakistan.

This type of work should be taken forward through both quantification and qualitative work. And quantification is an immediate priority. Somewhat surprisingly, despite the long history of the use of TMs, little is known about basic patterns of usage and such data is needed to provide a baseline from which to proceed to more complex studies of the processes surrounding provision and consumption. For instance, despite the extensive array of TMs currently available, and despite their export to the West, there is almost no data on consumption patterns in Pakistan's neighbour, India. While anecdotal evidence points to continuing extensive use, this needs to be tested empirically.

One of the issues raised by the Western sociology of CAM of relevance in this context is that of the relationship between the individual and the group. As suggested above, much has been debated in Western contexts regarding the relationship of the individual to their community or the state; notions of postmodernisation and late modernity have regularly been discussed in relation to changing patterns in healthcare consumption and behaviour. However, such questions have not been asked within the context of poorer countries. What is the relationship between community beliefs and individual decision making about therapeutic alternatives? To what extent are global changes towards the individual changing or reshaping decision making about local health practices? As such, there is a need for work that engages with the agency–structure dialectic in the context of poorer countries. This tension was highlighted in Chapter 8 as our work showed how the individual operates (somewhat precariously) at the intersection of the cultural and structural whilst also making individualised decisions.

Lastly, given the evident internationalisation of healthcare options, there is a need for investigation into the presence and potential role of non-indigenous CAMs in poorer countries like Pakistan. The theoretical possibility of their incorporation raises a number of questions. How will the entrance of non-biomedical globalised CAMs change (if at all) the relationship of TM and biomedicine? How will it impact on patients' decision making, and will consumption patterns be consistent with those seen in the West? And how will biomedical clinicians view CAM in the context of non-Western cultural contexts? The study of the potential three-way dynamic between indigenous TM, non-indigenous CAM and biomedicine will be central to the next stage of work.

The above, of course, merely represents a selection of the issues that need to be addressed. The key point is that a substantial sociological agenda awaits attention. While the pursuit of evidence driven by immediate policy demands will inevitably continue, an awareness of the need to address the use and provision of non-biomedical practices as a social process worthy of understanding in its own right should not be lost.

Notes

1 While we recognise the limitations of 'TM' as a category, and the wide range of practices that could come under its 'umbrella', we view it as a potentially useful generalised term that is also widely used by the World Health Organization.
2 The Prince of Wales's Foundation for Integrated Health was formed with the aim of encouraging complementary healthcare professions to develop and maintain systems of self-regulation. It also focuses on increasing the capacity for research into complementary medicine, and developing access to integrated healthcare.
3 Although prices can vary a great deal, the cost of going to see a (RSH) homeopath currently ranges from around £35–£95 for an initial consultation, and £20–£60 for follow-ups. Registered acupuncturists charge £15–£60, while a herbalist will cost around £40–£50 for a first consultation and £30 for a follow-up. Healing, reflexology and massage, etc. are generally cheaper, with one-to-one sessions starting from £15 (Pinder *et al.* 2005).
4 This particular therapist, after working as a healer within the NHS for over fifteen years, can legitimately claim to have been in the vanguard of integration, being one of the first individuals to be able to secure official funding for her activities.
5 Interestingly, it appeared that it was the therapist who found this background noise a problem. Very few of the patients who attended the group ever mentioned it. It seems that once they had been able to reach a certain state of relaxation, extraneous noise did not bother them. The therapist, on the other hand, was more acutely attuned to possible disturbance as she was guiding the session and remained in her normally conscious state.
6 This therapist, in common with many others who utilised spoken word-based approaches, produced material on CD and DVD which patients could listen to at home. These were essentially guided meditations very similar to those enacted during group sessions – the CDs were based on audio recordings of the therapist, and of two DVDs that had been produced, one was a full-length video of a 'live' session with the support group. The other was a short documentary which focused on de-mystifying the 'healing' process – a choice of subject which illustrates the degree to which she perceived her activities to be misunderstood. Demand for these recordings was reportedly very high, particularly among 'new' patients, or people who had little knowledge of what a group or one-to-one session would entail. They were distributed for free to anyone who expressed an interest.
7 Although we refer to people who attended the support group as 'members', there was no formal registration process. Arrangements were consciously informal and

although phone numbers of new members were sometimes taken, this was not done as a matter of routine.

8 An important element in the group sessions was the use of music. This was a ubiquitous backdrop to activities and was carefully chosen to enhance the atmosphere of relaxation that the therapist was intent on creating. The type of music used was surprising in the light of experiences in other CAM settings. Rather than the distinctive 'New Age' titles which are specifically produced to act as unobtrusive soundtracks to meditation activities, the therapist routinely played an eclectic mix of jazz and classical music – something which understandably produced polarised reactions from participants.

9 More than once, following particularly intense sessions, the therapist suggested to participants that they should avoid driving home straight away, and should make sure they were 'grounded' first.

10 A similarly difficult situation developed for the therapists running another one of our Type 2 groups. In this case, a new member joined who regarded herself as having far more therapeutic experience than the 'official' group leaders. Understandably, this created a tense and divided atmosphere at meetings for several weeks. Eventually matters came to a head and the individual decided to leave and start her own group – much to the relief of the organisers.

11 The material in the group library was rarely, if ever, accessed by medical staff, but its content was still sometimes a cause of concern for the therapist. On occasion, books had been donated which she thought might damage her already tenuous position within the hospital – should the staff find out she was giving them to patients. These included material on some of the more extreme dietary approaches to cancer management (which, she knew from past experience, the nutritionists working at the hospital were very much against), and books which basically encouraged patients to reject biomedical treatment. What is highly significant, however, is that the therapist maintained a private collection of 'extreme' books in a locked cupboard in her room (even going to the trouble of backing them with brown paper). These books were reserved for patients that she knew she could trust, and she affectionately called them 'my pornography collection'.

12 On one occasion that we were able to observe, a patient brought a jar of seeds to a meeting and was handing them around the group. She explained that she had bought them over the internet and that they were 'proven' to reduce the size of tumours. This understandably led to a discussion about whether this could be true or not, and soon the topic shifted to variations on conspiracy theories and the 'obstructive' behaviour of doctors. At this point, the therapist became involved and, perhaps surprisingly, made a persuasive argument supporting the role of biomedicine – even emphasising that remedies like this had not been tested in clinical trials. The fact that she did this when the mood of the group was becoming relatively militant (and thus, in a way, cohesive) demonstrated the priority she placed on expressing her neutrality. By adopting a more radical persona in this instance there would have been a clear potential for enhancing personal prestige within the group. That this was resisted is illustrative of the sensitivity to, and awareness of 'location' felt by her.

13 These are routinely 'healing', aromatherapy, massage and reflexology.

14 Taken from the Angel Hospice brochure.

Bibliography

Abbott, A. (1988) *The System of Professions: An Essay on the Division of Expert Labor*, Chicago: University of Chicago Press.

Adams, J. (2000) 'General practitioners, complementary therapies and evidence based medicine', *Complementary Therapies in Medicine*, 8: 248–52.

Ademsen, L. (2002) 'From victim to agent: the clinical and social significance of self-help group participation for people with life threatening diseases', *Scandinavian Journal of Caring Sciences*, 16: 224–31.

Alder, S. R. (1999) 'Complementary and alternative medicine use among women with breast cancer', *Medical Anthropology Quarterly*, 13(2): 212–22.

Bastien, J. (1987) 'Cross-cultural communication between doctors and peasants in Bolivia', *Social Science and Medicine*, 24(12): 1109–18.

Berman, B. M., Bausell, R. B. and Lee, W. L. (2002) 'Use and referral patterns for 22 complementary and alternative medical therapies by members of the American College of Rheumatology: results of a national survey', *Archives of Internal Medicine*, 162(7): 766–70.

Bishop, F. and Yardley, L. (2004) 'Constructing agency in treatment decisions: negotiating responsibility in cancer', *Health*, 8(4): 465–82.

Bodeker, G., Neumann, C., Lall, P. and Oo, Z. (2005) 'Traditional medicine use and healthworker training in a refugee setting at the Thai–Burma border', *Journal of Refugee Studies*, 18(1): 76–99.

Bodeker, G., Ong, C., Grundy, C., Burford, G. and Shein, K. (2005) *WHO Global Atlas of Traditional, Complementary and Alternative Medicine*, Kobe, Japan: World Health Organization Centre for Health Development.

Boon, H. (1998) 'Canadian naturopathic practitioners: holistic and scientific world views', *Social Science and Medicine*, 46(9): 1213–25.

Boon, H., Stewart, M., Kennard, M., Gray, R., Sawka, C., Brown, J., McWilliam, C., Gavin, A., Baron, R., Aaron, D. and Haines-Kamka, T. (2000) 'Use of complementary/alternative medicine by breast cancer survivors in Ontario: prevalence and perceptions', *Journal of Clinical Oncology*, 18(13): 2515–21.

Bourdieu, P. (1984) *Distinction: A Social Critique of the Judgement of Taste* [translated by Richard Nice], London: Routledge and Kegan Paul.

Briggs, C. L. (1989) *No Bones about Chiropractic? The Quest for Legitimacy by the Ontario Chiropractic Profession, 1895–1985*. PhD dissertation in Department of Behavioural Science/Community Health, University of Toronto, Toronto, Ontario, Canada.

British Medical Association (1993) *Complementary Medicine: New Approaches to Good Practice*, Oxford: Oxford University Press.

Broom, A. (2002) 'Contested territories: the construction of boundaries between "alternative" and "conventional" cancer treatments', *New Zealand Journal of Sociology*, 17: 215–34.

Broom, A. and Tovey, P. (forthcoming) *Therapeutic pluralism: Exploring the experiences of cancer patients and professionals*, London and New York: Routledge.

Calman, K. and Hine, D. (1995) *A Policy Framework for Commissioning Cancer Services*, London: Department of Health.

Cancerbackup (2001) *Directory of Cancer Services*, London: Cancerbackup.

Cancerlink (1998) *Directory of Cancer Self-help and Support*, London: Cancerlink.

Cant, S. and Sharma, U. (1996) *Complementary and Alternative Medicines: Knowledge in Practice*, London: Free Association Books.

Cassileth, B. and Chapman, C. (1996) 'Alternative and complementary cancer therapies', *Cancer*, 77(6): 1026–34.

Cassileth, B. and Vickers, A. (2005) 'High prevalence of complementary and alternative medicine use among cancer patients', *Journal of Clinical Oncology*, 23: 2590–2.

Chapman-Smith, D. (2001) 'Complementary and alternative medicine commonly used by cancer patients', *Medical Journal of Australia*, 175: 342–3.

Charmaz, K. (1990) '"Discovering" chronic illness: Using grounded theory', *Social Science and Medicine*, 30(11): 1161–72.

Chatwin. J, and Collins. S. (2002) 'Communication in the homoeopathic consultation', *The Homoeopath*, 84: 27–30.

Chatwin, J. and Tovey, P. (2004) 'Complementary and alternative medicine (CAM), cancer and group-based action: a critical review of the literature', *European Journal of Cancer Care*, 13: 210–18.

Coulter, I., Singh, B., Riley, D. and Der-Martirosian, C. (2005) 'Interprofessional referral patterns in an integrated medical system', *Journal of Manipulative Physiological Therapies*, 28(3): 170–4.

Coward, R. (1989) *The Whole Truth: The Myth of Alternative Health*, London: Faber.

CRUK (2006) UK Cancer Incidence Statistics, *Cancer Research UK*. Accessed online at: http://info.cancerresearchuk.org/cancerstats/incidence/

Damen, S., Mortelmans, D., and Van Hove, E. (2000) 'Self-help groups in Belgium: their place in the care network', *Sociology of Health and Illness*, 22: 331–48.

Department of Health (2000) *The NHS Cancer Plan – Making Progress*, UK: Department of Health.

Department of Health (2001) *The NHS Cancer Plan – Making Progress*, UK: Department of Health.

Dew, K. (1997) 'Limits on the utilization of alternative therapies by doctors: a problem of boundary maintenance', *Australian Journal of Social Issues*, 32(2): 181–97.

Dew, K. (2000a) 'Apostasy to orthodoxy: debates before a commission of inquiry into chiropractic', *Sociology of Health and Illness*, 22(3): 310–30.

Dew, K. (2000b) 'Deviant insiders: medical acupuncturists in New Zealand', *Social Science and Medicine*, 50(12): 1785–95.

Drew, P., Chatwin, J. and Collins, S. (2001) 'Conversation analysis: a method for research in healthcare professional-patient interaction', *Health Expectations*, 4(1): 58–71.

Eastwood, H. (2000) 'Postmodernisation, consumerism and the shift towards holistic health', *Journal of Sociology*, 36: 133–55.

Ernst, E. (2000) 'Unconventional cancer therapies', *Chest*, 117(2): 307–08.

Ernst, E. (2001) *The Desktop Guide to CAM*, Edinburgh: Mosby.

Ernst, E. (2004) 'Risks of herbal medicinal products', *Pharmacoepidemiology*, 13(11): 767–71.

Ernst, E. and Cassileth, S. (1998) 'The prevalence of complementary/alternative medicine in cancer: a systematic review', *Cancer*, 83: 777–82.

Eskinazi, D. (1998) 'Factors that shape alternative medicine', *Journal of the American Medical Association*, 280(18): 1621–9.

Featherstone, M. (1991) 'The body in consumer culture', in M. Hepworth and B. Turner (eds.) *The Body, Social Processes and Cultural Theory*, London: Sage.

Fulder, S. (1992) 'Alternative therapists in Britain', in M. Saks (ed.) *Alternative Medicine in Britain*, Oxford: Clarendon Press.

Fuller, R. (1989) *Alternative Medicine and American Religious Life*, London: Oxford University Press.

Fulton, G., Madden, C. and Minichiello, V. (1996) 'The construction of anticipatory grief', *Social Science and Medicine*, 43 (9): 1349–58.

Furnham, V. C. (1996) 'Why do patients turn to complementary medicine? An empirical study', *British Journal of Clinical Psychology*, 35: 37–48.

Gilbert, N. (1996) *Researching Social Life*, London: Sage.

Golomb, L. (1985) 'Curing and sociocultural separatism in South Thailand', *Social Science and Medicine*, 21(4); 463–8.

Gott, M., Stevens, T., Small, N. and Ahmedzai, S. H. (2002) 'Involving users, improving services: the example of cancer', *British Journal of Clinical Governance*, 7(2): 81–5.

Government of Lahore (2006) *Profile of Lahore*, Lahore: Government of Lahore. Accessed online at: http://www.lahore.gov.pk

Haram, L. (1991) 'Tswana medicine in interaction with biomedicine', *Social Science and Medicine*, 33(2): 167–75.

Harris, P., Finlay, I. G., Cook, A., Thomas, K. J. and Hood, K. (2003) 'Complementary and alternative medicine use by patients with cancer in Wales: a cross sectional survey', *Complementary Therapies in Medicine*, 11(4): 249–53.

Heritage, J. and Stivers, T. (1999) 'Online commentary in acute medical visits: a method of shaping patient expectations', *Social Science and Medicine*, 49: 1501–17.

Homedes, N., Ugalde A. and Chaumont, C. (2001) 'Scientific evaluations of interventions to improve the adequate use of pharmaceuticals in third world countries', *Public Health Reviews*, 29(2–4): 207–30.

House of Lords (2000) *Report on Complementary and Alternative Medicine*, London: House of Lords.

Hsiao, A., Ryan, G., Hays, R., Coulter I., Andersen, R. and Wenger, N. (2006) 'Variations in provider conceptions of integrative medicine', *Social Science and Medicine*, Jan 13 [epub ahead of print].

Iwu, M. and Gbodossou, E. (2000) 'The role of traditional medicine', *The Lancet*, 356, Suppl. s3.

Izzo, A., Di Carlo, G., Borrelli, F. and Ernst, E. (2005) 'Cardiovascular pharmacotherapy and herbal medicines: the risk of drug interaction', *International Journal of Cardiology*, 98(1): 1–14.

Johnson, J. and Lane, C. (1993) 'Role of support groups in cancer care', *Supportive Care in Cancer*, 1: 52–6.

Kelner, M. and Wellman, B. (1997) *Complementary and Alternative Medicine: Challenge and Change*, Amsterdam: Harwood Academic Publishers.

Khare, R. S. (1996) 'Dava, daktar, and dua: anthropology of practiced medicine in India', *Social Science and Medicine*, 43(5): 837–48.

Kohn, M. (1999) *Complementary Medicines in Cancer Care*, London: Macmillan.

Kronenfeld, J. J. and Wasner, C. (1982) 'The use of unorthodox therapies and marginal practitioners', *Social Science and Medicine*, 16: 1119–25.

Lewith, G., Broomfield, J. and Prescott, P. (2002) 'Complementary cancer care in Southampton: a survey of staff and patients', *Complementary Therapies in Medicine*, 10: 100–06.

Liede, A., Malik, I. A., Aziz, Z., de los Rios, P., Kwan, E. and Narod, S. A. (2002) 'Contribution of BRCA1 and BRCA2 mutations to breast and ovarian cancer in Pakistan', *American Journal of Human Genetics*, 71: 595–606.

Lindquist, G. (2001) 'The culture of charisma: wielding legitimacy in contemporary Russian healing', *Anthropology Today*, 17(2): 3–8.

Low, J. (2004) 'Managing safety and risk: the experiences of people with Parkinson's Disease who use alternative and complementary therapies', *Health* 8(4): 445–63.

Luff, D. and Thomas, K. (2000) 'Getting somewhere, feeling cared for: patient perspectives on CAM', *Complementary Therapies in Medicine*, 8: 253–9.

Lupton, D. and Tulloch, J. (2002) '"Risk is part of your life": risk epistemologies among a group of Australians', *Sociology*, 36(2): 317–35.

McClean, S. (2005) '"The illness is part of the person": discourses of blame, individual responsibility and individuation at a centre for spiritual healing in the north of England', *Sociology of Health & Illness*, 27(5): 628–48.

McGinnis, L. S. (1990) 'Alternative therapies: an overview', *Cancer*, 67: 1788–92.

MacLennan, A., Myers, S. and Taylor, A. (2006) 'The continuing use of complementary and alternative medicine in South Australia: costs and beliefs in 2004', *Medical Journal of Australia*, 184(1): 27–31.

Macmillan Cancer Relief (2002) *Directory of Complementary Therapy Services in UK Cancer Care: Public and Voluntary Sectors*, London. Macmillan Cancer Relief.

Malik, I., Kahn, N. and Kahn, W. (2000) 'Use of unconventional methods of therapy by cancer patients in Pakistan', *European Journal of Epidemiology*, 16: 155–60.

Michael, Y. L., Berkman, L. F., Colditz, G. A., Holmes, M. D. and Kawachi, I. (2002) 'Social networks and health-related quality of life in breast cancer survivors: a prospective study', *Journal of Psychosomatic Research*, 52: 285–93.

Micke, O., Mucke, R., Schonekaes, K. and Buntzel, J. (2003) 'Complementary and alternative medicine in radiotherapy patients – more harm than expected?', *International Journal of Radiation Oncology*, 57(4): 1197–8.

Miller, K. (1998) 'The evolution of professional identity: the case of osteopathic medicine', *Social Science and Medicine*, 47:11, 1739–48.

Miller, M., Boyer, M., Butow, P., Gattellari, M., Dunn, S. and Childs, A. (1998) 'The use of unproven methods of treatment by cancer patients: frequency, expectations and cost', *Supportive Care in Cancer*, 6(4): 337–47.

Montazeri, A., Jarvandi, S., Haghighat, S., Vahdani, M., Sajadian, A., Ebrahimi, M., and Haji-Mahmoodi, M. (2001) 'Anxiety and depression in breast cancer patients before and after participation in a cancer support group', *Patient Education and Counseling*, 45: 195–8.

Montbriand, M. (1998) 'Abandoning biomedicine for alternative therapies: oncology patients' stories', *Cancer Nurse*, 21, 36–45.

Morris, K., Johnston, N., Homer, L. and Walts, D. (2000) 'A comparison of complementary therapy use between breast cancer patients and patients with other primary tumour sites', *American Journal of Surgery*, 179(5): 407–11.

Mykhalovskiy, E. (2003) 'Evidence-based medicine: ambivalent reading and the clinical recontextualization of science', *Health*, 7(3): 331–52.

Napolitano, V. and Flores, G. (2003) 'Complementary medicine: cosmopolitan and popular knowledge, and transcultural translations – cases from urban Mexico', *Theory, Culture & Society*, 20(4): 79–95.

National Health and Medical Research Council (2005) *NHMRC Response to Senate Community Affairs References Committee Report the Cancer Journey: Informing Choice*, National Health and Medical Research Council.

Ngokwey, N. (1989) 'On the specificity of healing functions: a study of diagnosis in three faith healing institutions in Feira (Bahia, Brazil)', *Social Science and Medicine*, 29(4): 515–26.

Nigenda, G., Lockett, L., Manca, C. and Mora, G. (2001) 'Non-biomedical health-care practices in the State of Morelos, Mexico: analysis of emergent phenomenon', *Sociology of Health and Illness*, 23(1): 3–23.

Norris, P. (2001) 'How "we" are different from "them": occupational boundary maintenance in the treatment of musculo-skeletal problems', *Sociology of Health and Illness*, 23(1): 24–43.

Peace, G. and Manasse, A. (2002) 'The Cavendish Centre for integrated cancer care: assessment of patients' needs and responses', *Complementary Therapies in Medicine*, 10(1): 33–41.

Pinder, M., Pedro, L., Theodorou, G., Treacy, K. and Miller, W. (2005) *Complementary healthcare: A Guide for Patients*. London: Prince of Wales's Foundation for Integrated Health.

Pope, C. (2003) 'Resisting evidence: the study of evidence-based medicine as a contemporary social movement', *Health*, 7(3): 267–82.

Population Association of Pakistan (2002) *Pakistan's Population: Statistical Profile*, Islamabad: Population Association of Pakistan.

Rayner, L. and Easthope, G. (2001) 'Postmodern consumption and alternative medications', *Journal of Sociology*, 37(2): 157–76.

Rees, R., Feigel, I., Vickers, A., Zollman, C., McGurk, R. and Smith, C. (2000) 'Prevalence of complementary therapy use by women with breast cancer', *European Journal of Cancer*, 36: 1359–64.

Reissland, N. and Burghart, R. (1989) 'Active patients: the integration of modern and traditional obstetric practices in Nepal', *Social Science and Medicine*, 29(1): 43–52.

Research Council for Complementary Medicine (2000) *Survey of Knowledge and Understanding of Unconventional Medicine in Europe,* London: Research Council for Complementary Medicine.

Revil, J. (2002) 'Cancer sufferers warned off alternative measures', *The Observer,* 20 October.

Richardson, M., Sanders, T., Palmer, L., Greisinger, A. and Singletary, E. (2000) 'Complementary/alternative medicine use in a comprehensive cancer center and the implications for oncology', *Journal of Clinical Oncology,* 18(13): 2505–19.

Saks, M. (1998) 'Medicine and complementary medicine: challenge and change', in G. Scambler and P. Higgs (eds), *Modernity Medicine and Health,* London: Routledge.

Salmenpera, L. (2002) 'The use of complementary therapies among breast and prostate cancer patients in Finland', *European Journal of Cancer Care,* 11: 44–50.

Salmenpera, L., Suominen, T. and Lauri, S. (1998) 'Oncology nurses' attitudes towards alternative medicine', *Psycho-Oncology,* 7: 453–9.

Salminen, E., Bishop, M., Poussa, T., Drummond, R. and Salminen S. (2004) 'Dietary attitudes and changes as well as use of supplements and complementary therapies by Australian and Finnish women following the diagnosis of breast cancer', *European Journal of Clinical Nutrition,* 58(1): 137–44.

Scott, J. A., Kearney, N., Hummerston, S. and Molassiotis, A. (2005) 'Use of complementary and alternative medicine in patients with cancer: a UK survey', *European Journal of Oncology Nursing,* 29(2): 131–7.

Senate Community Affairs References Committee (2005) *The Cancer Journey: Informing Choice.* Commonwealth of Australia.

Sharma, U. (1993) 'Contextualizing alternative medicine: the exotic, the marginal and the perfectly mundane', *Anthropology Today,* 9(4): 15–18.

Sheldon, T. (2006) 'Dutch doctors suspended for use of complementary medicine', *British Medical Journal,* 332: 929.

Shuval, J., Mizrachi, N. and Smetannikov, E. (2002) 'Entering the well-guarded fortress: alternative practitioners in hospital settings', *Social Science and Medicine,* 55: 1745–55.

Siahpush, M. (1998) 'Postmodern values, dissatisfaction with conventional medicine and the popularity of alternative therapies', *Journal of Sociology,* 34: 58–70.

Siahpush, M. (1999) 'A critical review of the sociology of alternative medicine: research on users, practitioners and the orthodoxy', *Health,* 4(2): 159–78.

Sibbritt, D., Adams, J., Easthope, G. and Young A. (2003) 'Complementary and alternative medicine (CAM) use among elderly Australian women who have cancer', *Supportive Care in Cancer,* 11(8): 548–50.

Small, N. and Rhodes, P. (2000) *Too Ill to Talk? User Involvement in Palliative Care,* London: Routledge.

Sointu, E. (2006a) Recognition and the creation of wellbeing, *Sociology,* 40: 493–510.

Sointu, E. (2006b) The search for wellbeing in alternative and complementary health practices, *Sociology of Health and Illness,* 28(3): 330–49.

Sphere Project (2004) *Humanitarian Charter and Minimum Standards in Disaster Response,* Geneva: Sphere Project.

Stone, J. and Matthews, J. (1996) *Complementary Medicine and the Law,* Oxford University Press: Oxford.

Strauss, A. (1978) 'A social worlds perspective', *Studies in Symbolic Interaction,* 1: 199–228.

Targ, E. F. and Levine, E. G. (2002) 'The efficacy of a mind-body-spirit group for women with breast cancer: a randomised control trial', *General Hospital Psychiatry,* 24(4): 238–248.

Taveres, M. (2003) *National Guidelines for the Use of Complementary Therapies in Supportive and Palliative Care.* United Kingdom: The Prince of Wales's Foundation for Integrated Health.

The Cancer Council Australia (2006) 'Facts and figures', *The Cancer Council Australia.* Accessed online at: http://www.cancer.org.au

Thomas, K., Nicholl, J. and Coleman, P. (2001) 'Use and expenditure on complementary medicine in England', *Complementary Therapies in Medicine,* 9: 2–11.

Tovey, E. and Adams, A. (1999) 'The changing nature of nurses job satisfaction: an exploration of sources of satisfaction in the 1990s', *Journal of Advanced Nursing,* 30(1): 150–8.

Tovey, P. and Adams, J. (2001) 'Towards a sociology of CAM and nursing', *Complementary Therapies in Nursing and Midwifery,* 8(1): 12–6.

Tovey, P. and Adams, J. (2003) 'Nostalgic and nostophobic referencing and the authentication of nurses' use of complementary therapies', *Social Science & Medicine,* 56(7): 1469–80.

Tovey, P., Atkin, K. and Milewa, T. (2001) 'The individual and primary care: service user, reflexive choice maker and collective actor', *Critical Public Health,* 11(2): 153–66.

Tovey, P., Chatwin, J. and Ahmad, S. (2005) 'Toward an understanding of decision making on complementary and alternative medicine use in poorer countries: the case of cancer care in Pakistan', *Integrative Cancer Therapies,* 4(3): 236–41.

Tovey, P., Easthope, G. and Adams, J. (eds) (2003) *The Mainstreaming of CAM: Studies in the Social Context,* London: Routledge.

Turton, P. and Cooke, H. (2000) Meeting the needs of people with cancer for support and self-management, *Complementary Therapies in Nursing and Midwifery,* 6(3):130–7.

UNICEF (2006) *Pakistan at a Glance,* UNICEF. Accessed online at: http://www.unicef.org/infobycountry/pakistan_statistics.html

Urben, L. (1997) 'Self-help groups in palliative care', *European Journal of Palliative Care,* 4(1): 26–8.

Vincent, J. (1992) 'Self help groups and health care in contemporary Britain', in M. Saks (ed.), *Alternative Medicine in Britain,* Oxford: Clarendon.

Wayland, C. (2004) 'The failure of pharmaceuticals and the power of plants: medicinal discourse as a critique of modernity in the Amazon', *Social Science and Medicine,* 58: 2409–19.

Wheatley, C. (2002) 'Can fresh fruit really help you beat cancer?' *The Observer,* 15 September.

Whiteford, M. (1999) 'Homeopathic medicine in the city of Oaxaca, Mexico: patients' perspectives and observations', *Medical Anthropology Quarterly*, 13(1): 69–78.

WHO (World Health Organization) (2001) *Traditional Medicine Strategy 2002–2005*, Geneva: World Health Organization. Accessed online at: http://www.who.int/medicines/library/trm/trm_strat_eng.pdf

Zakar, M. (1998) 'Coexistence of indigenous and cosmopolitan medical systems in Pakistan', *International Public Health Series*, 1: 305.

Zollman, C. and Vickers, A. (1999) 'ABC of complementary medicine: users and practitioners of complementary medicine', *British Medical Journal*, 319: 836–8.

Index

Active engagement 6, 52, 102, 124, 134, 147
Aromatherapy and massage 18, 22, 34, 57, 66, 86
Australia, cancer 15–16, policy 19–20, case study 39–41, 100–113

Biomedicine 11–20; cost 135–7
Bourdieu, P. 139
Breast cancer 14, 17, 24, 96, 127; Pakistan 28, 119–122
Broom, A. 22, 61, 85, 131, 145–6, 164

Cancer: hospital 14–20; diagnosis 14–20; treatments 27; support groups 24–6, 50–1
Cancer Research UK (CRUK) 14–15
Cancer Council Australia, The 15–16
Cant, S. 16, 18, 20
Case study sites 33–6
Chemotherapy 53, 57, 64, 105
Complementary and alternative medicines (CAM) 12; definitions 11–14; policy 19–20; current use of 16–18; sociology of 20–4; support groups 24–6
Confined Innovation 81–99
Cost 29, 44, 59, 88, 130, 135–7
Cultural practices 138–41
Cure 18, 63–4, 129

Dam Darood 29, 119–29, 135–43, 150–7
Decision making: treatment 127; in support groups 23–6; pragmatic 137–8
Defining health practices 11–14
Department of Health 14–15, 19

Easthope, G. 21–2
Economic and Social Research Council 43
Education 28, 118, 122–3, 127
Effectiveness (patients' views) 123–6
Empowerment 25, 31, 63, 90, 94
Evidence 1–4, 59, 85, 117, 123–4, 146, 158–62 cancer; 14–16 anecdotal 14, in policy 19–20
Evidence-based medicine (EBM) 19, 123, 146
Expert knowledge 121

Faith 21, 128, 140–1, 163–4

General practitioners 124–5
Gerson Diet 58
Group performance 65–80

Hakeem 29, 120–2, 123–9, 138–41, 149–53
Healing 12, 18–19, 21, 25, 29, 35–6, 55, 57, 50
Healing Touch
Herbal Medicines 12, 17, 22, 30, 35, 56–7, 78, 119, 120
Holism 22, 31, 60–2, 86, 121, 149
Homeopath(s) 59, 125–6
Homeopathy 12–13, 18, 20, 30, 35, 57, 87, 94, 119, 120, 125
Hospitals 122–3
House of Lords 18
Hypnotherapy 19, 70

Identity 56, 90–2, 131, 134, 138–41
Inequality 94–8
Innovation 81–99, 101, 160
Integration 1, 12, 18–20, 23, 26, 58–9, 65, 85, 87, 91, 95–6, 98–9, 112

Internet 35, 36, 56, 96
Inter-professional issues 144–7;
    conflict 147–53; alliances 153–6
Islam 118, 128, 138–41, 153, 155

Lahore 41–3
Legitimacy 20–4, 30–1, 71, 133

Massage 12, 19, 34, 55, 57, 102
Medicalisation 50
Meditation 12, 33, 39, 40–1, 66, 70,
    73, 74–5, 76–7, 97–8, 101–13
Metaphysical 12–14, 67, 138–41, 142,
    149, 154, 157, 163
Methodology 32–45
Mind-body (medicine) 12
Morbidity (cancer) 14–16
Mortality (cancer) 14–16

National Health Service (NHS) 15, 18,
    19, 59, 70, 87, 91, 160
National Health and Medical Research
    Council (NHMRC) 19–20
Natural Healing 60, 69
Naturopath(y) 13, 17
Nurses/nursing 22, 57, 91

Orthodox medicine 11–12

Pain management 40, 62, 102, 110
Palliative care 16, 25, 102
Pakistan 38; cancer 28–9; use of TM
    119–21; fieldwork 41–4, 119
Pluralism 141–3, 156
Pirs 28–9, 149–53, 155–7
Policy (cancer) 19–20
Poorer countries 26–7

Postmodernisation 131, 165–6
Power/knowledge 20–4, 85–98
Professional boundaries 144–57
Professionalisation 13, 18, 20, 87, 95

Reflexology 19, 59, 86, 120
Reiki 11–13, 19, 51
Religiosity 138–41
Research Council for Complementary
    Medicine (RCCM) 18
Risk factors 14–15

Saks, M. 13
Satisfaction (levels) 123–6
Self reflection 63
Self-help groups 25–6, 49–50, 64, 84
Socioeconomic factors 129, 124
Spiritual healing 19, 25, 29, 63, 120,
    124, 136, 142, 155
Support groups 24–6; group types
    50–1; group evolution 53–66; group
    performance 65–80; CAM provision
    82–8; group innovation 88–94

Tovey, P. 20–4
Traditional healer(s) 30–1
Traditional medicines 26–7, 30–1; use
    in Pakistan 119–21; cost 135–7;
    accessibility 135–7

Wellbeing 56, 60, 128, 151
World Health Organisation 27, 117,
    144

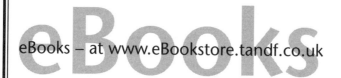